PELICAN BOOKS

A SACRED TRUST

Richard Harris, a staff writer at *The New Yorker* magazine
for the past fifteen years, has written extensively on politics. Among his works are the story of Senator Estes
Kefauver's attempts to regulate the pharmaceutical industry (*The Real Voice*—which prompted *Book Week* to
call Mr. Harris "the real voice of what American journal-
ism should be"), along with reports on such diverse
matters as the 1964 Republican Presidential Convention,
a Congressman's campaign for re-election, the struggle in
Congress and out over gun control, and the legislative
history of the Omnibus Crime Control and Safe Streets
Act of 1968.

A Sacred Trust

DISCARDED

RICHARD HARRIS

PENGUIN BOOKS INC

Penguin Books, Inc., 7110 Ambassador Road,
Baltimore, Maryland 21207, U.S.A.
Penguin Books Ltd, Harmondsworth,
Middlesex, England
Penguin Books Australia Ltd, Ringwood,
Victoria, Australia

First published by The New American Library, Inc. 1966
Published in Pelican Books 1969
Copyright © 1966 by Richard Harris
Copyright © 1969 Introduction by Edward M. Kennedy

Most of the contents of this book
appeared originally in *The New Yorker*,
in somewhat different form.

Set in Linotype Primer
Printed in the United States of America
by Universal Lithographers, Inc.

Introduction

SENATOR EDWARD M. KENNEDY

"ORDINARILY," Richard Harris says early in this narrative, "it takes a generation or more for Congress to approve a major piece of social legislation." That this generalization should be true is not any surprise to those of us who have served in the Congress, or worked in the Nation's capital; but this stubborn resistance to changing so many of our institutions comes as a continuing surprise to a great number of Americans all across the country. It is a contributing factor, I think, to the growing dissatisfaction with the unresponsiveness of the government as a whole—federal, state and local.

Mr. Harris masterfully details one specific case of this unresponsiveness—the resistance of the American Medical Association to Medicare. The battle for Medicare was one which actually raged for longer than a generation, as it was first introduced in the 1930's. The Medicare advocates won this battle in 1965 only in the face of determined, well-organized and well-financed opposition from the AMA. This case study is a fascinating insight into the legislative process as it had to confront this battle, for it mirrors the personalities of the principals and the mechanics of the process as it actually worked. It is this wealth of detail which makes *A Sacred Trust* as relevant today as when it was first published in 1966.

This book first appeared in somewhat different form in *The New Yorker* magazine, where the portrait it painted revealed to many Americans for the first time just how stubbornly the health profession resisted Medicare. When this portrait was expanded into its present book form, the case Mr. Harris presents becomes even stronger. And now that it is available in paperback form, and a larger audience has access to it, I would think that it might bring an even wider understanding of the frustrations of those Americans who recognize that changes are needed so badly, yet find it so difficult to bring them about.

We might do well to remember the context of the battle for Medicare. In his message to Congress transmitting the Medicare legislation, President Kennedy said:

"Illness strikes most often and with its greatest severity at the time in life when incomes are most limited; and millions of our older citizens cannot afford $35 a day in hospital costs. Half of the retired have almost no income other than their Social Security payments—averaging $70 a month per person—and they have little in the way of savings. One-third of the aged family units have less than $100 in liquid assets. One short hospital stay may be manageable for many older persons with the help of family and savings; but the second—and the average person can expect two or three hospital stays after age 65—may well mean destitution, public or private charity, or the alternative of suffering in silence. For these citizens, the miracles of medical science mean little."

The debate centered on the role of the government in lifting these senior citizens from lives of despair and pain. Today, we have difficulty understanding the intensity of the opposition to Medicare, because it has in its few years of operation brought so much to so many.

Our recent history is replete with other examples of these efforts at change being frustrated by institutional resistance. A most notable example is the need for gun control legislation. An overwhelming majority of Americans favored strict controls on the sale of guns—yet for years the effective lobbying opposition of the National Rifle Association kept these controls from ever appearing on our statute books. Last year, the Congress breached this previously solid front and passed a gun control law which imposes some mild controls; but they are filled with loopholes, and should be further strengthened.

There are many other examples as well. The oil import program has for years brought enormous windfalls to some oil companies in this country. The tax laws have made hundreds of "tax millionaires," while the low and middle-income taxpayers have had to bear a grossly distorted proportion of the tax load. The military-industrial complex has persuaded the Congress, in the name of national defense, to support programs for military hardware—programs full of waste, redundancy, and inefficiency. We have, for example, spent some $23 million on missiles deployed and then abandoned. Meanwhile, our schools and hospitals and housing programs have been starved for funds—while we have poured billions into road programs, farm subsidy programs, and other programs which make historical sense, perhaps, but not human sense.

One lesson the successful fight for Medicare teaches us is that institutions can be changed, even if the fight is long and painful. It took the prestige and commitment of President Kennedy, and later of President Johnson, as well as enormous public pressure, to win the Medicare fight. Partly as a result of this successful fight and a few others, there is a feeling spreading in this country that we should examine the underlying justifications for many of the multi-billion dollar federal spending programs. Many of these programs were designed years ago; many we extend year after year with only cursory independent discussions of their current relationships to a coherent, comprehensive set of national priorities.

There has recently been formed in the United States a Committee for National Health Insurance, under the chairmanship of Walter Reuther. The Committee seeks to develop a system of national health insurance to make comprehensive, high-quality personal health services available to every American, without reference to his income, his color, where he lives, or how old he is. There is a growing conviction that we have not matched the great advances in the medical sciences with health care programs which are truly relevant to the needs of our communities—all communities, and all citizens of these communities. The problems in undertaking to do so, of course, are complex and vast. They involve financing, organization of the health industry, the role of federal, state and local governments, nutrition, and many others. But just as the battle of Medicare was begun when only a few Americans knew the need existed and must be met, just so has a new battle been joined with the health institutions which will, more than likely, once again resist any change. We cannot now know the contours of the solution the Committee will propose; yet we know the problems need solution.

Hospital room rates are not $35 per day, as they were in 1963. They are now $65 per day. Drug costs have, in many cases, doubled in the last decade. Physicians fees have risen dramatically. In short, medical costs have taken an ever-larger share of the family budget. We must begin now to develop proposals to help families hard pressed by budget squeezes to meet their medical costs.

I think we can safely predict that the campaign for a system of national health insurance will not be a short one. We can also recognize the great needs—particularly among the poor in America, but equally among those middle-income Americans who watch with dismay the rapidly escalating costs of medical care. We are a great and rich nation, and there is hardly any rational explanation for our low standing in health care relative to the other advanced, industrialized nations of the world. We Americans have always prided ourselves on our ability to meet situations of difficulty or crisis with imagination and flexibility. The revolution of rising expectations—expectations which too often go unfulfilled—places us today in a crisis of a sort with which we are unfamiliar. It is not a threat to our security from an enemy intent on destroying us and our way of life. Rather, it is a threat to the fabric of our society, which is in danger of unravelling. We must meet this challenge, too, with imagination and flexibility, and not be wedded to the answers of yesterday.

A Sacred Trust tells us some of the reasons why it takes so long a time and such a commitment of energies to change a determined, entrenched institution.

If it takes us a generation each time in the future we set out to bring into effect a new piece of social legislation, we face very difficult times. Rereading Mr. Harris's book brings this clearly home.

Edward M. Kennedy
Washington, D.C.
March 20, 1969

SINCE the politician's first principle is to avoid taking on any more organized opposition than he has to, the first principle for those who want to influence politicians is to organize. With this elementary rule in mind, millions of people in the United States have banded together in some two thousand organizations and have sent their men off to Washington— lobbyists who represent everything from the National Association of Manufacturers and the American Federation of Labor-Congress of Industrial Organizations to the Camping Club of America and the Southwestern Peanut Shellers Association. For every member of Congress there are ten lobbyists, and the most modest estimates of what they spend in the course of working for or against specific pieces of legislation that interest their employers run to more than a billion dollars a year. In a sense, the Washington representatives of special-interest groups constitute a third house of Congress, since half of all the measures introduced in the Senate and the House of Representatives were originally written in their offices.

Far and away the most resolute contingent of lobbyists in recent years has been that of the American Medical Association. When the A.M.A. was founded, in 1847, its purpose, according to its constitution, was "to promote the science and art of medicine and the betterment of public health." Up until the time of the First World War, the Association restricted its activities to improving medical education, setting standards of practice, and policing quacks. Since that time, however, it has devoted more and more of its energies and considerable resources to persuading anyone who would listen, particularly lawmakers, that the only way to bring about the betterment of public health was to keep it in private hands. The dread of outside interference has led the A.M.A. to oppose even the mildest and most constructive official and semi-official intrusions, including compulsory inoculation against diphtheria and compulsory vaccination against smallpox, the mandatory reporting of tuberculosis cases to public-health agencies, the establishment of public venereal-disease clinics and of Red Cross blood banks, federal grants for medical-school construction and medical-student loans, Blue Cross and other private health-insurance programs, government subsidies to reduce maternal and infant deaths, and free centers for cancer diagnosis. The A.M.A.'s arguments against these proposals have ranged from charges that they constituted "bureaucratic interference with the sacred rights of the American home" to condemnation of them as "tending to promote Communism."

But the longest, bitterest, and costliest campaign the A.M.A. ever waged was its fight against any form of compulsory government health insurance, or what it has loosely called "socialized medicine." In that contest, like all the others, the A.M.A. possessed unique advantages. In 1964, for example, its total operating budget was twenty-three million dollars—or more than twice as much as that of its nearest rival, the A.F.L.-C.I.O. A large part of that sum paid for the upkeep of some nine hundred employees, including seventy publicists, at its headquarters in Chicago, as well as twenty-three members of its lobby office in Washington. Most of the Association's revenue came from advertisements in its various periodicals, but a full third of it was contributed in the form of dues by its two hundred thousand members—who possess some unique advantages, too. Among them are *their* incomes, which average out to the highest of any professional group in the country, and their prestige, which for many years survived even their own unwitting subversion of it. Politically speaking, these advantages are unmatched by any other lobby in the country. Even so, they scarcely compare to still another advantage with inestimable political potential—that doctors are practically ubiquitous; every day in every part of the coun-

2

try they can converse with, and possibly convert, some two and a half million patients.

The struggle over government health insurance raged back and forth across the country for more than a generation, it cost the A.M.A. and its affiliates and allies something on the order of fifty million dollars, it gave the Association a reputation that would not be envied by the Teamsters, and it left political wreckage that may not be cleared away for more than another generation. The long war finally ended in the summer of 1965 with enactment of the bill that is commonly known as Medicare—making the United States the last industrialized nation in the West to adopt a compulsory health-insurance program. When the bill passed, members of both political parties in both houses of Congress agreed that their votes on the measure were the most important ones that they had ever cast. "Medicare was the greatest social innovation since the passage of the original Social Security Act of 1935," Senator Clinton P. Anderson, Democrat of New Mexico, who was co-sponsor of the bill, said shortly after it passed. "The doctors claimed that the fight was over government control of medicine. That wasn't it at all. The fight was over whether decent medical care is a basic right—like the right to food, shelter, clothing, and education. The people and Congress decided that it was. I guess it could properly be called the fifth human right."

2

WHEN President Johnson flew to Independence, Missouri, on July 30, 1965, to sign the Medicare bill—officially designated Public Law 89-97—at the Harry S. Truman Memorial Library, he gave Mr. Truman credit for originating the legislation. Then he said, "We marvel not simply at the passage of this bill but what we marvel at is that it took so many years to pass it." While it is true that Mr. Truman was the first American President to make a public endorsement of compulsory health insurance, the idea was actually a good many years older than President Johnson indicated, and the new legislation had taken even longer to be passed. The idea originated, of all places, in Prussia when Bismarck, in 1883, instituted a medical-insurance plan, as a means of weakening trade unions and keeping the people beholden to the government— that is, to Bismarck. The idea of government medical insurance gradually spread through Europe, and in 1911 Great Britain set up a limited program to insure low-income groups against some of the high costs of sickness. The British program created interest in this country, and before it was a year old, Louis D. Brandeis, then a lawyer in private practice, urged the National Conference on Charities and Correction, a central organization made up of public and private welfare agencies, to support a broad program of social insurance, including medical insurance. His suggestion was accepted, and during the Presidential campaign of 1912 the Progressive Party, under Theodore Roosevelt, picked it up and made national health insurance one of the main planks in its platform.

That same year, the American Association for Labor Legislation—consisting of trade unionists, social reformers, economists, political scientists, and lawyers who had led the fight for state workmen's-compensation laws a few years earlier—set up a Committee on Social Insurance to try to devise a practical way of protecting the public against economically ruinous medical bills. (All in all, 1912 was a big year for medicine; according to an estimate made by Professor Lawrence Henderson, of Harvard, it also marked a significant dividing line in medical care—when "for the first time in human history, a random patient with a random disease consulting a doctor chosen at random stood better than a 50-50 chance of benefiting from the encounter.") In 1913, the Committee on Social Insurance reported back to its parent organization with a recommendation for a system of compulsory health insurance to be administered by the states. By 1915, the committee had drafted a model bill, and the following year several state legislatures began considering it seriously—and, for the most part, favorably.

The A.M.A. liked the idea, too, in those days. "The time has come when we can no longer resist the social movement, and it is better that we should initiate the necessary changes than have them forced on us," the trustees of the Association noted in a report on the subject of health-insurance coverage that was submitted to a meeting of the A.M.A. House of Delegates in 1916. Statements such as this one would be considered flagrant heresy a few years later, but in those days, when a long tradition of leadership by men like the Mayo brothers had made the A.M.A. into a universally respected scientific organization, sentiments of that sort did not seem unusual at all. Furthermore, the years just before the First World War in this country were a time of growing indignation against the brutal injustices of the industrial revolution, which were then being documented by writers like Lincoln Steffens and Upton Sinclair. Another A.M.A. statement of this period touched on the medical profession's concern and responsibility for the lot of the workingman: "The introduction of these [state health-insurance] bills marks the inauguration of a great movement which ought to result in an improvement in the health of the

5

industrial population and improve the conditions for medical service among the wage earners." The A.M.A.'s enlightened, if short-lived, view at that time reflected the influence of Dr. Alexander Lambert, Theodore Roosevelt's personal physician and a figure of great prestige within the medical profession. As chairman of the A.M.A.'s Social Insurance Committee, Dr. Lambert reported to the Association that his group had looked into the possibilities of voluntary health insurance under private control and, having found it unworkable, recommended adoption of a compulsory system under government control. The A.M.A.'s Council on Health and Public Instruction supported him. "Blind opposition, indignant repudiation, bitter denunciation of these laws is worse than useless," the Council informed the House of Delegates. "It leads nowhere and it leaves the profession in a position of helplessness if the rising tide of social development sweeps over [it]. . . . In the end the social forces that demand these laws and demand an improvement in the social existence of the great mass of the people of the nation will indignantly force a recalcitrant profession to accept." The A.M.A. delegates endorsed this prophetic statement without dissent, and by 1917 the model health-insurance bill had been introduced in sixteen state legislatures.

One of the earliest casualties of any war is social reform. When the United States entered the First World War, the health-insurance proposals, along with other remedial legislation, were shelved for the duration. Opponents of the idea, who turned out to be far more numerous than had been suspected, took the opportunity to group their forces. A great many doctors around the country—particularly practitioners in rural areas, who not only outnumbered their city colleagues but were in all ways more conservative—started writing letters to the *Journal* of the A.M.A. to express disapproval of the model bill. Their complaints—which were even more bitterly and persistently expressed on the local level—led county and state medical societies to send the A.M.A. official resolutions condemning its stand. Leaders in the pharmaceutical industry (who felt that government control over medicine would lead to government control over medication) and leaders in the insurance business (who felt that government health insurance would lead to government insurance of all kinds) joined the attack on government intervention. In the view of Frederic L. Hoffman, a vice-president of the Prudential Insurance Company of America and one of the chief spokesmen for the opposition, the whole health-insurance movement was clearly a German plot.

By 1920, the outcry against the model bill had become so clamorous that the A.M.A.'s House of Delegates reversed itself and passed a resolution declaring its "opposition to the institution of any plan embodying the system of compulsory contributory insurance against illness." Dr. Lambert was president of the Association that year, and during the session, a tumultuous one, delegates periodically broke into the chant "Get Lambert!" They got him by way of their resolution. That event marked a profound change in the A.M.A. Before long the great leaders in medicine—men like Lambert and the Mayos—disappeared for good from the Association's roster of officers. From that time on, the A.M.A. was largely run by what its detractors call "medical politicians." The 1920 resolution killed the model bill as far as the state legislatures were concerned, for these bodies had long since accepted organized medicine's authority in the field, and had, in effect, turned over to medical practitioners the final decision on all medical legislation. In the *laissez-faire* abandon of the twenties, few seemed to care.

If prosperity was the general rule of the twenties, no one had to look far for exceptions. Among millions weakened by impoverishment, thousands were dispatched each year, with terrifying regularity, by illnesses that they could not afford to have treated. Finally, a few people of influence who did care about the poor, including those who were made poor by medical bills, decided to do something about it. At their prompting, eight leading foundations got together in 1927 and set up a Committee on the Costs of Medical Care, consisting of prominent figures in the fields of medicine, public health, social work, education, and public affairs. Over a period of five years, the committee published twenty-eight reports, which constituted the most comprehensive survey of medical economics ever made up to that time. In 1932, the committee released its majority report, under the signature of its director, Dr. Ray Lyman Wilbur, a past president of the A.M.A. who had just served as Secretary of the Interior under President Hoover and at this time was president of Stanford University. Dr. Wilbur, and a majority of the committee's members, came out for group practice for doctors and voluntary health insurance for their patients.

The A.M.A. saw red. Commenting on the report, its *Journal* dismissed group practice as a system of "medical soviets," and then said, "The alignment is clear—on the one side, the forces representing the great foundations, public-health officialdom, social theory—even socialism and communism—inciting to revolution; on the other side, the organized medical profession of this country, urging an orderly evolution."

To the A.M.A., the alignment became clearer and clearer as time went on. Back in 1929, the program that was to become Blue Cross had been started in Texas—not so much to protect the patient against hospital costs as to protect hospitals against non-paying patients—and when the American Hospital Association endorsed the plan in 1933, the A.M.A. attacked it as a "half-baked scheme." The following year, the American College of Surgeons, one of the earliest organizations for specialists, announced its support for Blue Cross, whereupon the A.M.A. rebuked the surgeons for "an apparent attempt to dominate and control the nature of medical practice."

During Franklin D. Roosevelt's first term in office, it was clear that a large percentage of the American people were not just ill-fed, ill-clad, and ill-housed but also simply ill and unable to pay for medical care. Most charitable agencies, like practically everyone in those days, were short of funds, and they couldn't begin to cope with the medical needs of the millions who were out of work. In 1934, President Roosevelt appointed a Committee on Economic Security and assigned it the task of drawing up plans for a social-security system that

8

would give Americans some measure of protection "against misfortunes which cannot be wholly eliminated in this man-made world of ours." The committee recommended federal pensions, unemployment insurance, and direct assistance for certain categories of the needy, and suggested that an official study be made of the practicability of national health insurance. When the social-security bill came up before Congress the following year, it contained a sentence giving the Social Security Board, which was to administer the law if it passed, the power to make such a study and to report on it to Congress. According to the committee's staff director, Edwin Witte, "that little line was responsible for so many telegrams to the members of Congress that the entire social-security program seemed endangered." To save the program, the House Committee on Ways and Means, on orders from the White House, struck out the line.

Dr. John A. Kingsbury, a former Commissioner of Charities in New York City, attributed the protests to the A.M.A. and its state and county societies. "Like ordinary lobby groups they have sent thousands of telegrams to the President and to Congress, seeking to exert pressure without reference to the merits of the proposal under consideration," he said at the time. "They have sought to use personal influence on those in high places, have spent tens of thousands of dollars in publicity campaigns of misinformation, have spread false rumors, and have resorted to scurvy attack on personalities." Dr. Kingsbury soon had further reason to regret both the A.M.A.'s tactics and its influence. When he made his statement on lobbying, he was secretary of the Milbank Fund, one of the foundations that had underwritten the Committee on the Costs of Medical Care, and both he and the fund's chairman, Albert G. Milbank, who was also chairman of the Borden Company, were outspoken advocates of national health insurance. According to *Fortune,* "the connection between the Fund and the Borden Co. was made clear to the medical profession, and a number of local medical journals began hinting through editorials that a boycott of Borden products would have a salutary effect on the Fund." Shortly after the hinting began, the

9

Philadelphia Medical Roster & Digest was able to inform its readers that "one of the foundations has already modified its elaborate plan to sell state medicine for the simple but effective reason that many discerning physicians had stopped buying a certain product." The product was Borden's irradiated evaporated milk for infants. In March, 1935, Milbank announced that his fund did not endorse national health insurance after all, and not long after that Dr. Kingsbury was dismissed.

3

In POLITICS, a man who commands a consensus representing as much as two-thirds of his colleagues or his constituents in any given situation is looked upon with awe. If he has any percentage above that, people start muttering about tyranny. When the A.M.A. went into politics full time, beginning in 1935, its idea of a consensus among its members was that every single one of them had to support it all the time if their freedom was to be preserved. In an emergency session of the House of Delegates called early in 1935, while the social-security bill was pending before Congress, the A.M.A. again went on record against "all forms of compulsory sickness insurance." Two weeks later, to the astonishment of officials at the A.M.A. headquarters, in Chicago, the California Medical Association came out in favor of compulsory health insurance on the state level. After some pointed reminders from Chicago, the California doctors backed down. (In fact, they backed down so far that within a few years they were to spend a quarter of a million dollars to defeat the program they had previously endorsed.)

Then, in 1936, the federal government announced the findings of a two-year national-health survey, which showed that ninety per cent of the people in the country were getting inadequate medical care. In response to this survey, rebellion broke out in the A.M.A. itself. When the House of Delegates held its 1937 convention, the New York delegation submitted a resolution urging acceptance of the principle that "the health of the people is the direct concern of government," and advocating that the A.M.A. proceed to formulate a "national health policy." One observer noted that "hectic commotion

11

and violent waving of fists resulted," and the *Journal* reported that the proposal was "rejected with an enthusiastic unanimity."

Not all doctors were content to regard the matter as settled. A few months later, a group of four hundred and thirty internationally known specialists, deans of medical schools, and public-health officials formed a Committee of Physicians for the Improvement of Medical Care and issued a declaration that included most of the proposals the New York delegation had submitted to the House of Delegates. To meet this flank attack, an editorial in the *Journal* of the A.M.A. demanded that the signers of the declaration issue "prompt disclaimers" of their statement that the health of the people is the direct concern of government and went on to question the motives of some of them, naming names and suggesting that they were angling for government favors. At first, the members of the new committee had circulated their declaration only among doctors, but now they released it to the press. After that, the *Journal* refused to print articles or letters from any members of the committee.

The quarrel created lasting animosities, and drew a good deal of criticism on the A.M.A. from a number of the country's foremost physicians as well as from laymen. "Such methods of handling differing opinions coming from without, or dissent arising from within, are the tactics of sectarians, not of scientists," wrote Michael M. Davis, a well-known sociologist and medical administrator, who had been a leader of the health-insurance movement almost from its beginnings in this country. "They have had two unfortunate results. They have weakened confidence in the organized medical profession among considerable sections of the public. They have promoted among physicians an emotional approach to the economic and social aspects of medicine which warps and often inhibits an intelligent participation in problems in which the future of medicine is much involved." Actually, at that time doctors were far less united in their opposition to government participation in health matters than they came to be later. Polls showed that a majority of laymen supported national health insurance and that a majority of doctors agreed with them. Presumably, the two groups also agreed that more money should be available to pay for medical care. A study made several years before had shown that more than half the country's doctors had annual incomes of less than thirty-one hundred dollars. The A.M.A. had a solution for that problem, too—cut down on the number of doctors by restricting the number of students in medical schools, or what it called "professional birth control."

The A.M.A. found itself threatened by a second attack in 1937 that was in some ways far more serious. That year, several employees of the federal Home Owners' Loan Corporation, assisted by a few young New Deal attorneys, organized the Group Health Association of Washington, D.C. Their plan, designed for low-income government workers, was to hire doctors on a salary basis and to provide members with almost complete medical care for a monthly fee of two dollars and twenty cents apiece. Before the program got under way, the *Journal* warned doctors to stay clear of it, declaring, "Physicians who sell their services to an organization like Group Health Association for resale to patients are certain to lose professional status." Except for federal health insurance, nothing has alarmed organized medicine more than the idea of a group of people who want to pay their medical costs ahead of time getting together with a group of doctors who are willing to treat them for a stipulated monthly fee—an arrangement known as a prepaid group-health plan.

Back in 1929, Dr. Michael Shadid, a Syrian immigrant who had made a lot of money in private practice and wanted to share it, donated twenty thousand dollars to the Farmers Union Hospital Association, in Oklahoma, and, with its assistance, set up the nation's first medical coöperative, the Community Hospital-Clinic, at Elk City. The local medical society, which Dr. Shadid had belonged to for twenty years, tried to talk him out of going ahead. When that failed, it tried to expel him. When that, too, failed, the society disbanded and reorganized without him. After twenty years of harassment by the society, which refused membership to doctors participating in the program, the clinic finally sued the society for three hundred thousand dollars, charging restraint of trade. Eventually the society settled out of court, and agreed to admit the proscribed doctors to membership.

The A.M.A.'s case against prepaid group-health plans has been essentially the same as its case against health insurance. Both grew out of a "statement of principles" that the House of Delegates adopted in 1934 which asserted, among other things, that "no third party must be permitted to come between the patient and his physician in any medical relation." In much of its literature, the A.M.A. has referred to this as "the sacred doctor-patient relationship"—or, if it is feeling uneasy, as "the sacred patient-doctor relationship." Whatever it is called, an almost magical quality has been assigned to it. There is no doubt that a patient's belief in his doctor's powers has often been the best medicine available to either of them. Few potions in the old-fashioned country doctor's little black bag had as much effect as his kindly demeanor and his comforting hands.

To an extent, faith in one's doctor is still sometimes vital. As Bronislaw Malinowski, the famous anthropologist, has written, "Magical beliefs and practices tend to cluster about situations where there is an important uncertainty factor and where there are strong emotional interests in the success of action." Aside from religious practices, probably no human situation fits this description better than that of a person undergoing medical treatment. "The basic function of magic," according to Talcott Parsons, professor of sociology at Harvard, "is to bolster the self-confidence of actors in situations where energy and skill *do* make a difference but where, because of uncertainty factors, outcomes cannot be guaranteed. This fits the situation of the doctor, but in addition on the side of the patient it may be argued that *belief* in the possibility of recovery is an important factor in it. . . . Of course, this argument must not be pressed too far."

No one has pressed the argument further than the leaders of the A.M.A., who have used it as their chief argument against any interference with the intimacy of a doctor's re-

14

lationship with his patient. Advocates of government health insurance have argued that the only relationship it necessarily interferes with is the one between a patient and his pocketbook. Moreover, some of them have pointed out, it was in the depths of the Depression that the A.M.A. adopted its "statement of principles," and in those days a relationship with any doctor outside a charity ward was a luxury that not many Americans could afford. Various developments in medicine since then have diminished the intimacy of the relationship still further. Thirty years ago, for example, the average doctor treated perhaps fifty patients a week, and now the number has trebled. Moreover, the rapid growth of specialization (today there are some fifty specialties and subspecialties) has cut the number of family doctors from one for every nine hundred people to one for every three thousand. In sum, the average patient nowadays gets less of his doctor's time than a patient did in the thirties, and is more likely to be sent on to a specialist, whom he may never have seen before. Should his illness require that he be sent to a hospital—the time when he most needs the security of such a relationship —a host of third parties, including internes, residents, nurses, orderlies, technicians, are bound to come between him and his doctor.

Regrettable as the loss of personal attention may be, the scientific advances that have taken its place seem—to many people, at any rate—a worthy substitute. Selig Greenberg, a journalist and medical writer, has pointed out that there is a certain irony in the A.M.A.'s defense of the inviolability of that relationship, since it has consistently encouraged the kind of modern medical practice that makes it less and less attainable. In Greenberg's view, "all the befuddlement of inane oratory cannot quite obscure the fact that the medical profession is using the largely mythical rapport between doctors and patients as a weapon in the battle to protect its lucrative privileges."

On the subject of how doctors should be paid, the A.M.A. has been uncompromising. The 1934 "statement of principles" stipulated that "however the cost of medical service may

15

be distributed, the immediate cost should be borne by the patient . . . at the time the service is rendered." In further support of what is known in medical circles as the "fee-for-service" doctrine, the House of Delegates later passed a resolution stating, "Any system of medicine that offers complete coverage and relieves the recipient of making any direct contribution for his own medical care will lower his sense of responsibility for his own health and that of his family and will eventually depreciate the quality of medical services he receives." In substance, the fee-for-service doctrine means that only a doctor can determine what his services are worth.

To critics like Greenberg, the doctor-patient relationship is sacred to doctors largely because it keeps outsiders from comparing or questioning fees. Another well-known medical writer, Richard Carter, has claimed that the A.M.A.'s opposition to any large-scale health-insurance program "has been based on the fear that economic plans of that scope would require public support so extensive as to necessitate public control." And he continued, "The knowledge that public control will curtail the profession's fee privileges underlies organized medicine's position on health insurance and on every other controversial issue in the field."

The A.M.A. has also often spoken of the virtues of "free-enterprise medicine." In a sense, it is the purest form of free enterprise, because under it every doctor is an individual entrepreneur—entirely free to practice as he sees fit and to charge what he wants. At the same time, the A.M.A. quietly opposes what it calls "corporate medicine," which, despite its ominous sound, means merely that a doctor chooses to work for a salary, whether on the faculty of a medical school, in a research foundation, at a hospital, in government service, or in private industry. The proportion of salaried physicians in this country has risen in the past thirty years from about a seventh to better than a third, so the A.M.A. has done no more than hint that this means of earning a living is unethical. However, it has not attempted to stop some county medical societies from expelling members who accept salaries.

The pressures on doctors who defy any of the A.M.A.'s

basic precepts have often been severe. By 1938, the Group Health Association of Washington had enrolled twenty-five hundred members and their dependents, who were taken care of by seven doctors working on salary. The group was small, but the fact that it was run by and for government employees added to its importance as a precedent. At first, the A.M.A. appealed to the seven doctors to withdraw from the program. When they refused, the District of Columbia Medical Society sent all its members a so-called white list of approved organizations that they could belong to. The Group Health Association was not among them. When the seven doctors still refused to give up their salaried group practice, they found that they were no longer being called in for consultations and that referrals of patients, the staple of specialty practice, abruptly stopped. Still they stuck it out. The District society then persuaded most of the hospitals in the area to deny staff privileges to the rebels and beds to their patients. One doctor who had taken a woman patient to a hospital for surgery and had already given her morphine was suddenly refused access to the operating room; after a four-hour quarrel with the hospital director he moved his patient to another hospital. A man with acute appendicitis was dismayed to learn that his own doctor would not be permitted to operate on him, and that the operation would not be performed at all unless he agreed to withdraw from the program. One stubborn old woman who had been run over by an automobile was finally forced to leave the hospital to which she had been rushed because she persistently refused to be treated by anyone but a Group Health Association doctor.

Just when the doctors in the program were about to admit defeat, Thurman Arnold, the chief of the Antitrust Division of the Department of Justice, heard about what was going on and sent out some investigators to collect evidence, which he then presented to a grand jury. The A.M.A. and the District of Columbia Medical Society were indicted for violation of the Sherman Antitrust Act. The government lost the case in a lower court but won a reversal in a higher court and made it stick in the Supreme Court. In a unanimous decision, written

17

by Justice Owen J. Roberts, the Court held that the A.M.A. was guilty of a criminal action, and went on to say:

> Professions exist because people believe they will be better served by licensing specially prepared experts to minister to their needs. The licensed monopolies which professions enjoy constitute in themselves severe restraints upon competition. But they are restraints which depend upon capacity and training, not privilege. Neither do they justify concerted criminal action to prevent the people from developing new methods of serving their needs. The people give the privilege of professional monopoly and the people may take it away.

The government had won its case against the A.M.A. because it had been able to prove that a conspiracy existed. And it had been able to prove that a conspiracy existed because the A.M.A. hadn't bothered to conceal it. Afterward, the A.M.A. continued to oppose prepaid group-health and insurance plans but employed somewhat different tactics. "Recently, organized medicine has conveyed veiled threats to doctors participating in disapproved plans by outspoken condemnation of such plans in ethical terms," the *Yale Law Journal* commented several years after the Court's decision. "Such indirect, less overt opposition probably discourages physicians from affiliating with disapproved plans, but is less susceptible to antitrust prosecution." Indirect methods were apparently enough to do the job, for the article added, "Defiance of A.M.A. authority means professional suicide for the majority."

Nor was there any way for most of the victims of reprisals to fight back. Courts invariably ruled that expulsion from, or denial of membership in, a county medical society—often entailing a loss of hospital privileges and specialty accreditation, which could mean the loss of a doctor's practice—did not deprive a doctor of any property right, and as long as the society didn't violate its own rules, they rarely intervened; that is, unless a society ignored the Supreme Court decision and excluded a member for participating in a group-health plan. Ultimately, then, nonconformists were pretty much at the mercy of their

18

colleagues. "The doctor who challenges A.M.A. authority to determine his method of practice," the *Yale Law Journal* noted, "is tried and judged by his fellow physicians who may have an economic interest in proscribing his allegedly offensive conduct."

4

No ONE except its own officers has ever cited the A.M.A. as a model of the democratic institution. In theory, its structure is democratic, but in practice it stifles just about any dissension within the ranks. At the bottom are roughly two thousand county medical societies, whose members elect not only their officers but representatives to state societies. Similarly, the members of the state societies elect not only their officers but representatives to the national House of Delegates. In both county and state societies, however, the presiding officer appoints a committee to nominate all candidates, and a rigid tradition of professional dignity rules out electioneering. It would be difficult to devise a more effective arrangement for guaranteeing that every elected official will tend to agree with every other elected official.

The national House of Delegates names the A.M.A.'s board of trustees, its annual president, and several other national officers. The delegates are supposed to set A.M.A. policy, at meetings held twice a year, but they usually approve what the trustees recommend. (Whenever an unacceptable resolution is submitted, the speaker of the House turns it over to a reference committee, whose members he has appointed.) The president of the A.M.A. has great prestige within the organization but not much power. The men who actually run things are the executive vice-president and his assistant, both of whom are also doctors. For the most part, they stay out of the limelight as they guide the Association in its everyday operation, which in the long run determines its direction. Another way that the A.M.A. preserves its monolithic character is by seeing to it that dissenters have no effective way to dissent. Nothing in the by-laws prevents delegates from making all the protests they want to. But the sort of man who becomes a delegate— typically, a small-town specialist with an interest in medical politics and time on his hands whose views on matters of policy have been checked at each upward step—is disinclined to fight with headquarters, so anyone who wants a scrap usually finds himself quickly voted down. Neither the *Journal* nor the *AMA News* (a weekly tabloid) is known to favor manuscripts and letters that diverge from official policy.

Yet all these bricks in the A.M.A.'s façade might come tumbling down if it weren't for the mortar holding them together —the background and attitude of the doctors who support the Association. The doctors who *don't* support it—mainly those practicing in large cities, the more accomplished specialists and researchers, and teachers in medical schools—are not typical of the profession as a whole. (They usually avoid challenging the A.M.A., because any dispute with it can be dangerous and is bound to be futile.) One explanation of the general unanimity among doctors lies in the well-documented fact that most physicians are highly educated within their field and almost not at all outside it. According to Milton Mayer, the essayist and social critic, "A doctor is, by definition, a man who doesn't have time. One of the things the average doctor doesn't have time to do is catch up with the things he didn't learn in school, and one of the things he didn't learn in school is the nature of human society, its purpose, its history, and its needs. . . . If medicine is necessarily a mystery to the average layman, nearly everything else is necessarily a mystery to the average doctor."

Most doctors began specializing in the natural sciences in their mid-teens, and, aside from browsing through some required courses in general studies, they specialize for the rest of their lives. Unless they happen to be outstandingly gifted, they have to, if they hope to keep up at all with medicine's prodigious growth. The exacting demands of medical school, the duration of the necessary apprenticeship, and the time spent in learning about the latest developments have produced what is sometimes called "the Cadillac syndrome." One

21

physician who looks at this development with alarm has said, "After all, a doctor goes through a fearful grind, living close to poverty, before he gets established—usually not until his mid- or late thirties. It's small wonder that by the time he does, he's determined to resist any threat to his income." A study made by E. Lowell Kelly, a professor of psychology at the University of Michigan, indicated that this attitude tends to appear even before the fearful grind has begun—among medical-school applicants, in fact. "Essentially, our medical students are . . . not the kind of people who would become teachers, ministers, social workers, i.e., professional persons interested in doing something for the good of mankind," Professor Kelly reported. "As a group, the medical students reveal remarkably little interest in the welfare of human beings. . . . It is my impression that the typical young executive in big industry today has a far greater sense of community needs and sensitivity to his role in helping society solve its problems than does the young physician."

A few years ago, Richard Carter visited the A.M.A.'s Chicago office and interviewed the top men. "During my visit to A.M.A. headquarters, I was flabbergasted to hear how many leading Republicans are regarded there as 'doctrinaire Socialists,' " he wrote later. "I finally solved the puzzle by realizing that the A.M.A. believes its own propaganda." With increasing insistence since the nineteen-thirties, that propaganda has centered on the phrase "socialized medicine," which the A.M.A. has never actually defined but which has been endlessly repeated until it has become what Carter calls a "patriotic malediction." Whatever else the campaign against socialized medicine may have done, it has certainly succeeded in scaring the wits out of the A.M.A.'s members. In the thirties, before the campaign really got under way, a majority of doctors favored government health insurance; today nine out of ten doctors are against it.

The person who is generally given most of the credit for this remarkable conversion is Dr. Morris Fishbein, who was the editor of the *Journal* and the A.M.A.'s chief spokesman— indeed, its *de-facto* leader—throughout the nineteen-thirties and forties. Dr. Fishbein joined the A.M.A. staff, as assistant to the editor of the *Journal,* in 1913, a year after he graduated from Rush Medical College, in Chicago. From the start he devoted most of his waking hours and his burning energy to the cause of warning his colleagues about the looming spectre of socialized medicine. It was he who expanded and consolidated the A.M.A.'s powers, kept the rank-and-file in line with a hint here and a threat there, and—most notable of all—turned out the huge amount of publicity about government meddling in medicine. In 1938, *Fortune* described Dr. Fishbein as "a promoter," and commented, "He has promoted the A.M.A. from a mild academic body into a powerful trade association." In the process, Dr. Fishbein became so closely identified with the group he spoke for that it was often referred to by detractors as the American Fishbein Association.

Not long after *Fortune*'s appraisal appeared, Dr. Fishbein got a chance to test the power of his trade association on a national scale. Back in 1935, President Roosevelt had appointed an Interdepartmental Committee to Coördinate Health and Welfare Activities, and after three years of work the committee submitted its report, entitled "A National Health Program," to a National Health Conference that was conducted under Presidential auspices in 1938. The report recommended that government participation in the field of public health be greatly increased, to include, among other things, federal health insurance, and, over the animated opposition of the A.M.A.'s representatives at the meeting, it was endorsed by the conferees. On February 28, 1939, Senator Robert F. Wagner, Sr., of New York, introduced a measure—he called it the National Health Bill—that translated the health-insurance part of the report into legislative language. The bill provided for federal grants to match state allocations for public-health programs, as long as they were approved by the Social Security Board and offered "services and supplies necessary for the prevention, diagnosis, and treatment of illness and disability." Wagner's estimate of his plan's cost to the federal government in its first year of operation was thirty-five million dollars.

When Roosevelt announced that he supported the Wagner bill, the A.M.A. hurriedly sent some of its officials to the White House to remind him that they opposed compulsory government health insurance. Ignoring Wagner's protest that his bill did "not establish a system of health insurance or require the states to" and was therefore not compulsory, the A.M.A. charged that it provided for "supreme federal control" over medicine and would lead, "insidiously," to "a complete system of tax-supported governmental medical care." As Dr. Fishbein described the bill, in a speech before the American Association for Social Security, it was "another step toward the breakdown of American democracy." Most of his listeners were social workers, who were less alarmed than disappointed by the bill, because they knew that most of the states were unable to put up much money for medical care, however generously it might be matched. Dr. Fishbein diverted his audience further by telling them that the inability of the poor to obtain medical services was not a problem for the medical profession but one for social workers, who had "failed miserably" in that regard.

The National Health Bill struck most people as a fairly innocuous measure; it appeared, stated the New York *Times,* "to face only minor opposition in the Congress." Alerted by this assessment, the A.M.A. called a war council in Chicago, and a few months later the House of Delegates, meeting in St. Louis, adopted a "declaration of principles" that stated, among other things, that the A.M.A. was "unmistakably and emphatically" opposed to the Wagner bill as "a threat to the national health." The day after the delegates voted on the measure, the Association's president-elect, Dr. Nathan B. Van Etten, called for all-out war against the Wagner bill. He gave the delegates specific instructions on how to wage the war:

Every delegate must realize his official obligations as never before and carry home to every single practitioner in his state a full consciousness of the importance of this declaration of principles. That practitioner is potentially one of the most powerful persons in the democracy. If he can be made to see his duty to his country and educate his patients to a realization of the dangers of centralized control of medical practice, your action of yesterday will be sustained.

The sanctity of the doctor-patient relationship, it appeared, was to be sacrificed to political expediency. Being able to issue warnings of political danger to people already feeling endangered by illness was an advantage that no politician on the other side could hope to match. "It is in the very nature of illness that it impels the individual back toward his childhood and even beyond," Dr. Flanders Dunbar has written in her book "Mind and Body," a standard work on psychosomatic medicine. "This is especially true of his emotional reactions. He wants to be taken care of, to have the burden of decisions taken from his shoulders, to be protected and cherished." Under these conditions, it would not be difficult for a doctor to convince a patient that if government health insurance were to be enacted, he would never be protected and cherished again.

Still another tactical innovation came out of the war council in Chicago. This was the founding of the National Physicians' Committee for the Extension of Medical Service (whose actual purpose was to keep medical service exactly as it was). The A.M.A. claimed that it had nothing to do with the new outfit—the N.P.C., as it was called—but the chairman of the N.P.C. was a past president of the A.M.A., the executive board of the N.P.C. included three members of the A.M.A.'s board of trustees, the secretary of the N.P.C. was the secretary of the A.M.A., and the N.P.C.'s money was provided by the A.M.A.'s fund-raising apparatus. Dr. John P. Peters, a professor at the Yale School of Medicine and a spokesman for the Committee of Physicians for the Improvement of Medical Care (whose actual purpose was to improve the A.M.A.), charged that the N.P.C. was designed "to serve as a cloak for lobbying activities" of the A.M.A. Casting off its cloak at the very start, the N.P.C. announced in its first press release that it was "primarily an instrument of propaganda" and that it hoped to "make enough noise so that congressmen will find some other

25

worm besides 'free medical care' with which to feed their peeping constituents." When word got out that Dr. Fishbein was sitting in on the N.P.C.'s strategy meetings, it was clear that the A.M.A. had gone into politics in a big way.

In politics, the appearance of power is often as useful as its reality—as long as no one challenges it. Once the A.M.A. had embarked on a political career, its leaders were convinced that they had power to spare, and so were many members of Congress. But to a large extent the Association's power was an illusion—one whose existence depended on the politician's characteristic reluctance to get involved in any test of strength that might show his own power to be illusory. In any event, the legend of invincibility that the A.M.A. built up over the years began in 1939, when the Wagner bill unexpectedly died in committee. Out in Chicago, the A.M.A. congratulated itself on having quashed the "grandiose scheme," and in Washington people began to look upon the A.M.A. with increased respect.

Actually, the credit should have gone to President Roosevelt. Perhaps his thoughts about running for a third term made him reluctant to push for any controversial program, however popular, at that particular moment. Or perhaps he had in mind the Presidential, or Vice-Presidential, prospects of another candidate, Paul V. McNutt, who, not entirely to Roosevelt's liking, was gaining support in the Party. As Federal Security Administrator, McNutt was the administration's chief spokesman for the Wagner bill, and its passage would have added considerably to his prestige. Whatever the reason, just before Christmas of 1939 the President withdrew his endorsement of the bill, on the ground that the program was too costly, and the measure was put aside.

5

AFTER the attack on Pearl Harbor, it seemed unlikely that any new domestic social-welfare legislation would be passed for some time. The war itself, though, soon raised some important questions about American medical care. For one thing, the number of young men who were unfit for military service, often because of physical defects that proper care could have prevented or corrected, proved to be alarmingly high. And then the millions of men who *were* fit grew accustomed to the fact that they could always see a doctor when they were sick —a new experience for many of them. A poll conducted by *Fortune* in 1942 showed that 74.3 per cent of the people favored national health insurance. At this point, Senator Wagner decided to try again. Along with Senator James E. Murray, Democrat of Montana, and Representative John D. Dingell, Sr., Democrat of Michigan, he submitted, in June of 1943, the first of a series of similar measures—known as the Wagner-Murray-Dingell bills—that were to be introduced off and on in Congress over the next fourteen years. This first one, which was far more ambitious than the 1939 bill, called for comprehensive medical, hospital, dental, and nursing-home care for almost everyone in the country. The care was to be paid for out of a special fund built up from equal contributions by employers and employees.

Although Representative Dingell had high hopes for the bill and believed that it would be enacted within a few years, Senators Wagner and Murray were convinced that nothing would come of it so soon. However, the two senators had been quick to agree to sponsor the measure when it was described to them by the men who were largely responsible for drafting it—Wilbur Cohen and I. S. Falk, both of the Social Security Board. "Senator Wagner heard us out and, after five minutes' discussion, gave us his O.K.," Cohen recalled not long ago. "He didn't have to know what was in the bill, word for word, because he knew that it would never be passed in anything like its original form, or, for that matter, in *any* form, for a good many years. But he also knew that something of the sort would go through ultimately, and he wanted to start things moving. Back in 1930, when he introduced a federal unemployment-compensation bill, everyone told him that he was crazy and that it would never get anywhere. Well, it became law in 1935. This was the same sort of thing for him—a long-range plan." As for Senator Murray, he was of much the same mind, although he felt that there would be some earlier, indirect effects from the bill. "Murray knew that the A.M.A. would kick up a hell of a fuss about it, which was exactly what he wanted," William Reidy, the Senator's assistant for many years, remarked recently. "He planned on letting the doctors publicize the measure for him, and then, once the public was aroused, to get bits and pieces of the original enacted as separate legislation. In effect, that's exactly what happened."

Dr. Fishbein reacted as Murray had predicted he would. Calling the bill "a blue-print for medical revolution, dealing with the sick and with the physicians who care for them as inanimate units to be moved at a dictator's will," he went on to say that the proposal was "perhaps the most virulent scheme ever to be conjured out of the mind of man." Even this language was not strong enough for some doctors. While they retained their membership in the A.M.A. for practical reasons, they set up their own militant organization, the Association of American Physicians and Surgeons. Its first official act was to pledge a boycott not only of the bill, if it should be enacted, but of any doctor who spoke out in favor of it in the meantime.

No one knew exactly how much the Wagner-Murray-Dingell program would cost—no one, that is, except organized medicine's "instrument of propaganda," the N.P.C., which distributed fifteen million copies of a pamphlet entitled "Abolishing Private Medical Practice, or $3,048,000,000 of Political Medicine Yearly in the United States." The issue, according to the N.P.C.'s pamphlet, was "human rights as opposed to State slavery." The forms of slavery it claimed would be visited upon the public included a government plan to pay doctors only for an eight-hour day, with the result that evening emergency cases would have to wait until morning; a plan to allow "bureaucrats" to decide which doctor a patient went to; and a plan to forbid doctors to make any medical decisions without first consulting more "bureaucrats." Another product of the N.P.C. campaign was a poster cartoon designed for display in doctors' waiting rooms. It showed an elderly woman timidly facing a wrathful doctor (or perhaps it was a wrathful bureaucrat in doctor's clothing) who was saying, "Make it snappy, sister." The text explained, "The doctor can't sit listening to your tale of woe. He's not a private physician. He works for the government, not you. You're just one of the people assigned to him by the political overseer. . . . So snap into it, comrade!"

No bill has ever been introduced in Congress to force doctors into being government employees—except, of course, the draft law. The Wagner-Murray-Dingell bill specifically provided that physicians could refuse to treat any patient for any reason, or could stay out of the program altogether, and that patients could choose to be treated by any doctor who participated. It did stipulate that fees would be subject to government regulation. In any event, the measure died in committee; once again Roosevelt was in the process of deciding whether to run for another term.

Shortly after the 1944 election, the President apparently decided that the time had come for action on national health insurance. Summoning a group of experts, he told them to draft a Health Message to be sent to Congress—the first message of its kind. He wanted it to suggest various improvements in the field of public health, he said, but primarily he meant to use it to persuade Congress to enact something along the lines of the Wagner-Murray-Dingell bill. Taking on a pressure group like the A.M.A. before the election was one thing, but taking it on afterward was quite another. "He was clearly looking forward to doing battle with those fellows in Chicago," one of the experts he summoned recalled not long ago. "He seemed amused by their political pretensions." But President Roosevelt never got his chance to match wits with the A.M.A.; before the message was completed, he died. Those who had been working on the document concluded that it had died with him. Most of them considered the new President a rather conservative man, and, in any event, they felt he had enough on his hands. They took their preliminary drafts of the message to the White House as a matter of course, and, to their surprise, Mr. Truman said it was a fine idea. He added, however, that it would have to wait until the war was over.

The wait wasn't a long one. Three months after V-J day, President Truman sent the message to Congress. In an attempt to ward off the old ritual charges of socialized medicine, he took pains to define the limitations he wanted to see written into any health-insurance bill. "People should remain free to choose their own physicians and hospitals," he said, and added, "Likewise, physicians should remain free to accept or reject patients. They must be allowed to decide for themselves whether they wish to participate in the health-insurance system full time, part time, or not at all." The N.P.C. didn't see the situation that way. "Authority is to be given a single government official to hire doctors . . . to control and operate hospitals . . . and to conduct the business of peddling pink pills to people," it announced. Cohen and Falk prepared a new bill, and Wagner, Murray, and Dingell, with the administration's blessing, filed it in the Senate and the House. The passage of such a bill, according to the *Journal*, would "mean the end of freedom for all classes of Americans." And Dr. Fishbein told the N.P.C., "No one will ever convince the physicians of the United States that the Wagner-Murray-Dingell bill is not socialized medicine." Adding that the President's message concealed an "insidious strategy," and that the bill would create "the kind of regimentation that led to totalitarianism in Germany," he called on his listeners to defeat it "ignominiously."

6

To THOSE who produced A.M.A. literature—and to many of those who read it—the federal government had by this time come to seem like a ravening wolf, threatening to devour all those who took upon themselves the business of caring for the sick—or what the medical profession often calls "a sacred trust." State governments, on the other hand, had generally been viewed as docile lambs, and could be counted on to show proper respect for the doctors' prerogatives. But in 1945 California revealed that it had a pretty fair set of fangs of its own. Late that winter, Governor Earl Warren surprised the medical profession by sending a compulsory health-insurance bill to the state legislature. The California Medical Association had proposed an almost identical program ten years before, but now it recoiled in alarm. Encouraged by the A.M.A., it quickly armed itself for a fight to the finish.

To meet this new threat of "socialized medicine"—a term that Governor Warren called an "ideological blackjack"—the California Medical Association hired a local public-relations firm called Whitaker & Baxter, which was the first in the country to specialize in politics. The founders of the firm, Clem Whitaker and Leone Baxter, his wife, held that old-fashioned lobbying—persuading, intimidating, and buying legislators—was costly and, in the long run, uncertain, since a client could not be sure that legislators would stay persuaded, intimidated, or bought beyond a single legislative session, and the whole unpleasant business might have to be repeated every couple of years. Whitaker & Baxter operated on the principle that a far better approach was to convince the voters of the worth of any given cause and let *them* do the arm-twisting, at election time. Lawmakers could thereby be kept in line longer, without endless campaign contributions and the other expenses of influence. The expenditure of money for public rather than private persuasion had been a common practice among business groups since at least the nineteen-twenties, but Whitaker liked to trace his professional lineage back to Lincoln, who once said, "Public sentiment is everything. With public sentiment, nothing can fail; without it, nothing can succeed."

Whitaker & Baxter's first move was to devise an alternative to compulsory health insurance, for, Whitaker solemnly told the doctors, "you can't beat something with nothing." His solution was to drum up support for Blue Cross, Blue Shield, and commercial health-insurance plans—that is, to make an issue out of voluntary versus compulsory health insurance. The over-all campaign was divided into a number of operations, which were carried on more or less simultaneously. The firm set out to get the principle of voluntary insurance endorsed by local and state organizations of all kinds, and within three months it had signed up more than a hundred groups that carried political weight. A speakers' bureau was organized, and before long nine thousand doctors, armed with speeches written in what Whitaker & Baxter called "fighting prose," were out on the stump. As an additional precaution, the firm engaged in some straightforward lobbying by sending doctors and influential friends to drop in for chats with the principal backers of the state's hundred and twenty assemblymen and senators. Physicians also visited the heads of four hundred service clubs, two hundred and eighty officers of veterans' groups, five hundred officers of women's clubs, two hundred insurance executives, and officials of every state, county, city, and town agency of any size.

But the most important and carefully planned approach was the one made to the press. One of Whitaker & Baxter's subsidiaries was the California Feature Service, a weekly sheet of political news and more or less unobtrusive plugs for the firm's clients, which was sent free to all the small newspapers in the state. About three hundred of them, mostly weeklies that were short on staff and funds, used the material regularly, either rewritten in the form of editorials and columns or, sometimes, verbatim. As the campaign against the Warren bill increased in momentum, a large part of the sheet's news was made up of attacks on the bill. In addition, Whitaker later reported to California doctors, "Our people have personally called at more than five hundred newspaper offices, talking doctors' problems with the editors, placing copy with them, and urging them to make your battle their battle." He was able to point to impressive results: the number of papers in the state opposing the bill soon rose from about a hundred to four hundred and thirty-two. Of course, the callers from Whitaker & Baxter were not the only forces of persuasion that newspaper publishers and editors encountered during that period. In an article that later appeared in the *Journal* of the A.M.A., the secretary of the California Medical Association mentioned another factor that may have played a part:

> At present the California Medical Association is spending $100,000 a year in newspaper advertising. . . . Never before have we been able to get real support from the newspapers because the answer constantly came back, "Why should we give the doctors any support when they don't advertise . . . ?" We now have an answer to that. When we started our campaign, we went to the California Newspaper Publisher's Association and said, "Gentlemen, we are going to spend a lot of money with the newspapers. We are going to advertise in every one of the 700 newspapers in California. . . ." We have found the response from editors, in publicity, has been beyond anything we expected when we started the campaign.

In three months, doctors and businessmen friendly to their cause purchased seventy thousand inches of advertising space in California papers. The Warren bill was defeated.

The entire campaign had cost the California Medical Association a quarter of a million dollars. It also cost the medical profession a certain amount of good will. Increasing numbers of people, in California and elsewhere, were finding it difficult

33

to believe that doctors would spend all that money just to protect their patients. And millions of people who were living on limited incomes were becoming more and more disturbed about the rapidly rising costs of medical care, which in many cases were pricing that precious commodity out of their reach. "It seemed to many of us at the time of the fight against the Warren bill that the doctors were in danger of drowning in the flood of their own invective," one of President Truman's advisers on health matters recalled recently. "The people wanted the best that medicine had to offer. If it was too expensive for most of them—well, then, they were bound to demand help in paying for it. All the bombast in the world couldn't stop them from getting what they felt they had a right to."

Sensing the growing public antagonism to the doctors' stand, the A.M.A. turned for advice to another public-relations firm, Raymond Rich Associates, of New York, and ordered a thorough appraisal of its non-medical activities. Many of the Association's critics, especially doctors in academic life, were dismayed by this move, suspecting that one public-relations firm would be bound—by professional ethics, if not by self-interest—to give nothing but a hearty endorsement to a course of treatment that had been prescribed by another public-relations firm. However, after a lengthy study Raymond Rich Associates turned in a report recommending that the N.P.C. be disbanded, or at least sharply curtailed; that the research data the A.M.A. published to prove its political case be substantiated; and that the A.M.A. set up some kind of a forum through which dissenters could have their say. The leaders of the A.M.A. were as stunned as everyone else. They rejected the recommendations and refused to make any changes. At that point, the Rich firm tendered its resignation and mailed copies of it to all members of Congress. "The Association," the letter read, ". . . has yet to seek the truth on the economic and social aspects of medicine, to put the public first, and to become adequate to its responsibilities."

7

ORDINARILY, it takes a generation or more for Congress to approve a major piece of social legislation. Even when the legislators are favorably disposed toward such a bill, it faces what one political commentator has called "a stupefying amount of discussion"—hearings in committees of the Senate and the House, debate on the floor of both chambers, debate in the press, debate among the public at large, and then still more hearings and still more debate in Congress. Except for periods of national emergency, anything controversial is bound to be handled cautiously on Capitol Hill, and in the late nineteen-forties Congress was certainly not in a rash mood. With the greatest war in history just ended, members of Congress seemed to want a breather, a chance to look around. Aside from the Wagner-Murray-Dingell bill's inherently controversial nature, quite a few men in government had misgivings about particular features of it—about its magnitude, for one thing. After all, they pointed out, the Depression was past, the majority of the people were fairly well off, and the growth of both commercial and nonprofit health insurance was proceeding at a promising rate. Maybe something more modest would suffice, they felt.

In 1946, Senator Robert A. Taft, the leader of the conservative coalition in Congress, moved to solve the problem once and for all by introducing a bill that would provide matching grants to states for medical care for all those who could pass a means test proving that they were indigent. He was jumped on from all sides. William Green, president of the American Federation of Labor, testified at the hearings on the measure, "The workers of this country are not prepared to accept the pauper oath as the approach to better health." The Committee of Physicians for the Improvement of Medical Care, which was still trying to improve the A.M.A., denounced it as a shoddy attempt "to relieve physicians of the burden of charitable services rather than to insure to patients more and better care." And the A.M.A. said it amounted to socialized medicine.

The following year, Wagner, Murray, and Dingell once more gamely submitted their bill, and once more hearings were held, and once more nothing came of them. As before, President Truman supported the proposal and was attacked by the A.M.A.—this time for claiming that only three and a half million Americans had adequate health-insurance protection. Dr. Fishbein himself stated that only a million people were covered—an unexplained decline from an estimate of five million that he had made in 1943. The chairman of the A.M.A.'s board of trustees took issue with both men; the correct number, he said, was fifty-five million.

Like any negotiator, a politician who proposes a new law ordinarily asks for more than he expects to get, in the hope that by trading a horse here and rolling a log there—always in a spirit of judicious compromise—he will end up with what he was willing to settle for in the first place. The process demands special prudence and skill, particularly in an election year. On January 7, 1948, President Truman told Congress in his State of the Union Address, "This great nation cannot afford to allow its citizens to suffer needlessly from the lack of proper medical care," and asked it to enact "a comprehensive insurance system to protect all our people equally against . . . ill-health." The Wagner-Murray-Dingell bill was still before Congress, but no one outside the A.M.A. had any illusions about its chances. For one thing, it had never got anywhere when the Democrats controlled Congress, and now the Republicans were firmly in command of both houses. Furthermore, there is nothing that members of Congress care less for than having to take a stand on a hotly debated subject just before facing the voters. In this instance the conservatives didn't want to stir up the labor unions, and the liberals didn't want to stir up the doctors and their allies.

No matter how deeply Mr. Truman believed in the Wagner-Murray-Dingell bill, it seemed clear to many people at the time that he also found it handy as a club with which to belabor the "do-nothing Eightieth Congress." The strategy helped him, but it didn't help the cause of government health insurance at all. By asking for far more than anyone imagined Congress would give him, he made it certain that he would get nothing. And by turning health insurance into a campaign issue rather than working quietly for it in the usual way—through persuasion and pressure on the Hill—he created a mood of cynicism among members of Congress on both sides of the aisle. During the campaign, Mr. Truman spent so much time defending the bill and attacking its opponents that the cynicism began to spread throughout the country.

The A.M.A. quickly came to the President's rescue. Its spokesmen travelled around the country making fiery speeches in which they charged that Mr. Truman was an avowed Socialist who was hellbent on destroying American freedom. The effect was that public interest revived, and so, in time, did public indignation. Commenting on the A.M.A.'s claim that enactment of the bill would destroy at one stroke all that the country stood for, Milton Mayer wrote in *Harper's,* "A nation's liberties would seem to depend upon headier and heartier attributes than the liberty to die without medical care." An editorial in *Life* noted, "The ever-rising costs of medical care and how to lessen them, if possible, are problems of national concern. But the [A.M.A.] seems to be against almost anything that threatens the profits of a doctor's private practice. It is not against the invaluable doctor but against medicine's official spokesman that great sections of our people have turned as bitter as they were against bankers during the Depression." The bitterness increased when the N.P.C. placed an advertisement in *Editor & Publisher* that February announcing a contest, with three thousand dollars in prizes, for the best "published" cartoons portraying "the

37

meaning and implications of 'political distribution of health care services in the United States.' " In the following issue, *Editor & Publisher* stated editorially, "The 'contest' rules leave no doubt that this is a subtle bribe to cartoonists to support or oppose certain political beliefs . . . and to obtain general circulation for those beliefs in newspapers and magazines."

Undeterred by the furor that the contest had caused, the N.P.C. proceeded to send a letter to all the country's doctors and clergymen—or, at least, all who were Christians. Described by the N.P.C. as "one of the few really vital pronouncements of an age," the letter started out "Dear Christian American," and went on to imply that certain non-Christians, whom it didn't identify, were leading the fight for socialized medicine. And the reader was warned to be prepared for the inevitable results of national health insurance—free love, birth control, and a dangerously high birth rate. The letter was signed "Reverend Dan Gilbert." In addition to being the editor of an extreme-rightist magazine called the *Defender*, Gilbert had been closely associated with the pro-Nazi Silver Shirts before the war. When the letter and Gilbert were described in the press, the A.M.A. quickly disavowed any connection with either of them. By the end of that year, the N.P.C. had spent, in all, more than a million dollars. It had apparently also spent whatever public prestige remained to it, for shortly afterward it was disbanded.

8

PRESIDENT TRUMAN's victory in the 1948 election was so narrow that to many people it seemed he had been given little more than the authority to remain in office. Although members of his party on the ticket regained control of Congress, their margin was slim, too, and a coalition of Southern Democrats and Northern Republicans ran both houses, as it had before. To the A.M.A., however, the election results meant that socialized medicine was about to become the law of the land. A month after the election, the House of Delegates convened in St. Louis in what one participant called "a spirit of great urgency." In a closed session, one speaker said, "Within a period of months, a crisis will have to be met. This is not a mere statement—it is an incredible reality." It certainly would have seemed incredible to the administration. By then, Mr. Truman had privately conceded that there was no hope of getting anything like the Wagner-Murray-Dingell bill through Congress and had told his staff to look around for something more promising. The unions, having come to the same conclusion, had turned their attention to collective bargaining as the second-best way to get health protection for their members.

In the opinion of some observers, the A.M.A.'s panic had been deliberately created by a handful of its top officers, who saw an opportunity to enlarge their own powers. This opinion gained wider acceptance when the board of trustees resolved that each A.M.A. member be assessed twenty-five dollars to create a three-and-a-half-million-dollar "war chest," which would be used to organize "the greatest grass-roots lobby in history." Although the A.M.A. had never imposed any form of dues in the hundred years of its existence, the delegates approved the resolution with little debate. Payment was to be voluntary the first year (nearly two-thirds of the members volunteered, quite a few of them after Dr. George Lull, the Association's secretary, announced that in the event of resistance "appropriate disciplinary action will be taken"), but it was to be mandatory from then on.

The assessment was widely criticized. The Lobby Investigating Committee of the House of Representatives called it "blatant, undisguised coercion." G. Bromley Oxnam, a bishop of the Methodist Church and a member of the Committee for the Nation's Health, which had been established in 1946 in New York, said, "The assessment put upon every American doctor to raise a propaganda fund that today is being used to misinform a nation is a national disgrace." In the medical world, more than a hundred eminent physicians got together and signed a protest stating that the assessment would "add to the already firmly rooted suspicion that the Association's objectives are primarily economic and selfish." Many less eminent doctors were reluctant to speak out that frankly. As Dr. Ernst P. Boas, chairman of a small and more or less heretical group called the Physicians' Forum, pointed out in a letter to the *Times*, the A.M.A. was not a private club that one could easily resign from. "Membership is almost indispensable to the practicing physician, because many privileges and opportunities such as hospital appointments and admissions to examination by the specialty boards are largely contingent on such membership," he explained. One man who decided that his membership was dispensable, whatever the cost, was Dr. James Howard Means, chief of medical services at the Massachusetts General Hospital, professor at the Harvard Medical School, and former president of the American College of Physicians; in resigning, he announced that he could not go on "supporting an activity . . . contrary to public welfare and unworthy of a learned profession."

The A.M.A. did not take this kind of criticism lying down. One of the physicians who had signed the protest against the assessment was notified by the Arkansas State Health Office that his appointment as a consultant to the Arkansas State Board of Health was being withdrawn because of his action. The A.M.A. called the Physicians' Forum a Communist front. The *Journal* refused to print an advertisement for an issue of the *Atlantic* that contained an article by Dr. Means. And the president of the A.M.A., in a column that appeared in the *Journal,* told his readers, "The pinkish pigmentation (and that's a mild way of saying it!) of the Committee for the Nation's Health—many of whose officers, directors and most vocal members have been listed in the files of the House Un-American Activities Committee for subversive connections or activities—should give you new assurance of the rightness of your cause when that committee violently attacks you." Besides Bishop Oxnam, the officers of the committee included Robert F. Wagner, Jr., Philip Murray, John Gunther, Arthur Goldberg, William Green, Robert E. Sherwood, Abe Fortas, and Mrs. Eleanor Roosevelt.

Perhaps the most objective comment on the whole question of the assessment was provided by Oscar Ewing, who served as Federal Security Administrator under President Truman. When asked about the A.M.A.'s new tactic, he said, "If their cause is good, they don't need three and a half dollars. And if their cause is no good, ten times three and a half million dollars won't enable them to fool the American people."

Although the A.M.A. had stated that its new funds were to be spent not on lobbying but on "stimulation," one of the first things it used the money for was to hire more lobbyists for its office in Washington. All the big decisions, however, were to be made in Chicago. (The men in Washington spent much of their time warning the head office about what was happening, or was likely to happen, in the capital, and spent the rest of their time putting out political fires that were lighted by the Chicago headquarters after their advice was ignored.) The bulk of the assessment was allocated to what was called a National Education Campaign. Everyone assumed that the campaign would be headed by Dr. Fishbein, but this time the trustees passed over Dr. Fishbein in favor of the firm of Whitaker & Baxter, which they retained at a fee of a hundred thousand dollars a year. "The p.-r. fellows have been Rasputin to the medical profession's czar," Nelson Cruikshank, the social-security director of the A.F.L.-C.I.O., remarked not long ago. "Ever since that first fat fee Whitaker & Baxter got, the rest of them have been trying to scare hell out of the A.M.A. It's been rumored that they've even planted health-insurance bills in Congress, and then have run to the A.M.A. with surefire plans for defeating them."

Some doctors were dismayed not only by the choice of campaign managers but by the campaign itself. One of them—Dr. Thomas S. Mattingly, a prominent physician in Washington, D.C., who said he had followed the debate over the Warren bill with "a sense of fascinated revulsion"—told the press that although Whitaker's chief talent was for "the suffocating cliché," apparently the A.M.A. had convinced itself that "Oscar Ewing would never socialize medicine so long as Whitaker & Baxter had three million dollars to spend on tracts, holy relics, and pictures."

Whitaker & Baxter set up an office in Chicago, staffed it with thirty-seven assistants, and announced that it would put on a "factual and dignified" campaign. By the time President Truman delivered his State of the Union Address in January of 1949, and once more came out for the Wagner-Murray-Dingell bill, Whitaker & Baxter was ready for him. "We will offer a positive program," Whitaker announced, "because we realize that you can't beat something with nothing." The positive program, like the reason given for offering it, turned out to be identical with the one that Whitaker & Baxter had persuaded the California Medical Association to accept in order to defeat the Warren bill—voluntary health insurance. "This brings the A.M.A. up to being only twenty years behind the times," one member of Congress said. The A.M.A. did not make the advance without difficulty. To accept Whitaker's program, it had to disown one of the most compelling arguments ever made against voluntary health insurance, which was published by its own Bureau of Medical Economics back in 1934. After deploring any form of compulsion in health-insurance matters, the bureau's report stated, "Without some

form of compulsion, voluntary insurance fails of its objective
of distributing the cost of sickness among large classes of the
population with even approximate fairness. The young and
healthy will not join and the aged and sickly, if accepted, will
raise the cost to a prohibitive point and, if rejected, [will]
remove protection from those most in need." But when the
A.M.A. embraced voluntary health insurance in 1949, it also
claimed that it had been one of the first supporters of the idea.
The claim was not widely honored. An article that appeared
in *Medical Economics*, a far from radical magazine, observed
that "the doctrinaire view crediting the A.M.A. with early
sponsorship of experimental voluntary prepayment programs
emerges as a simple untruth." *Hospitals*, the official publication of the American Hospital Association, declared in an editorial, "It is a sad fact that through the 1930's and early
1940's the American Medical Association did not believe in
voluntary sickness insurance, and did almost everything possible to prevent its development."

One of the pieces of literature most widely distributed during Whitaker & Baxter's National Education Campaign was a
fifteen-page question-and-answer pamphlet entitled "The Voluntary Way Is the American Way." A sampling of its contents
gives the flavor of the entire campaign:

Q. Who is for Compulsory Health Insurance?
A. The Federal Security Administration. The President. All who seriously believe in a Socialistic State.
Every leftwing organization in America. . . . The Communist Party.

Q. What is "compulsory" about Compulsory Health Insurance?
A. The payroll tax is compulsory. There is no es-
cape from it. But there is no compulsion on Government to . . . fulfill promises. That's the joker!

Q. How much will the tax be?
A. Sponsors have used various figures. Estimates
range from 3% to 10% on every paycheck up to $4,800.
[The government's highest estimate was four per cent,
and the maximum taxable amount was not a paycheck
of $4,800 but an annual income of $4,800.]

Q. Why should the cost, even for second-rate service, run so high?

A. . . . America would require a million and a half non-medical employees—clerks, administrators, book-keepers and tax-collectors—on the Federal payroll, si-phoning off medical funds before they ever bought the patient care of any kind. [That year, the number of civil-ian employees in the entire executive branch of the fed-eral government was 1,702,377.]

Q. Where did Compulsory Health Insurance start?

A. Germany had the first and strongest all-inclusive program. If the world needs proof of what regimentation and political domination of doctors and scientists can do, even in this modern world—the Nuremberg Trials have supplied it. [Bismarck was not a defendant at Nu-remberg.]

Q. Under Compulsory Health Insurance, may a pa-tient choose his own doctor?

A. . . . There is no guarantee of freedom of choice. [The Wagner-Murray-Dingell bill guaranteed free choice.] . . . Proponents of Compulsory Health Insurance in this country promise that patients would be free to choose their own doctors. But this same promise was made in England. It is an empty promise, never kept. [Under Brit-ain's National Health Service program, which went into effect in 1948, patients were able to choose their own doctors; they still are.]

Q. Would socialized medicine lead to socialization of other phases of American life?

A. Lenin thought so. He declared: "Socialized medi-cine is the keystone to the arch of the Socialist State." [The research staff of the Library of Congress has never been able to find this quotation, or anything like it, in Lenin's works.]

Whitaker & Baxter was said to be especially proud of an-other product of the National Education Campaign—a repro-duction of Sir Luke Fildes's famous painting "The Doctor." The picture, which dates from the eighteen-forties, shows a doctor sitting, head in hand, beside a small girl on a make-shift bed of pillows on two chairs; the father is standing help-lessly beside her, and the mother, her head down on a nearby table, is either sobbing or sleeping. Whitaker & Baxter had seventy thousand posters made up with the Fildes painting above this caption:

KEEP POLITICS OUT OF THIS PICTURE!
When the life—or health of a loved one is at stake, hope lies in the devoted service of your Doctor. Would you change this picture?
Compulsory health insurance is political medicine.
It would bring a third party—a politician—between you and your Doctor. It would bind up your family's health in red tape. It would result in heavy payroll taxes —and inferior medical care for you and your family. Don't let that happen here!

Dr. Means, of the Harvard Medical School, observing that anyone in his right mind certainly *would* change this picture, pointed out that Fildes's doctor was clearly not much better equipped to help the child than her parents were, and that under modern conditions she would be in a hospital, where a whole battery of third parties would come between the family and their doctor in order to save her life. A more appropriate title, he said, would have been "Keep This Picture Out of Medicine." Anachronism or not, the poster appeared in thousands of doctors' waiting rooms around the country. Before the year was out, Whitaker & Baxter had produced over forty other posters, plus pamphlets, leaflets, folders, booklets, cards, and cartoons, and had distributed, by its own count, 54,233,915 of them, at a cost of $1,045,614.52.

All this promotional material, while it was noisy enough to attract a good deal of attention, was only the small-arms fire of the campaign. For the big thrust, Whitaker & Baxter brought up its heavy artillery—endorsement of the A.M.A.'s position by medical, paramedical, and, most important, non-medical organizations throughout the country. Tactically, the support was made to appear the result of spontaneous indignation over what the government proposed to do. Form speeches were sent to all state and county medical societies, accompanied not only by specific instructions on where, when, and how they should be delivered but by lists of various

45

groups in each region, noting who their officers were, when they met, and what kinds of audiences they could be expected to provide. The firm also sent each local medical society a batch of form resolutions that its speakers were to have endorsed by the organizations they addressed. Once an endorsement was obtained, copies were to be sent to the state governor and legislators, to members of Congress, and to the President. After that, the local society was to prepare press releases announcing the endorsement, and to deliver them to all newspapers and radio stations in the immediate area.

By the end of 1949, Whitaker & Baxter had lined up eighteen hundred and twenty-nine organizations behind the A.M.A., including the Daughters of the American Revolution, the National Association of Retail Grocers, the United States Chamber of Commerce, the American Council of Christian Churches, the General Federation of Women's Clubs, the National Grange, the American Legion, the National Conference of Catholic Charities, the American Bar Association, and the American Farm Bureau Federation, along with such less well-known but equally staunch supporters as the Trailer Coach Manufacturers Association, the American Institute of Laundering, the National Plywood Distributors Association, and the Toastmasters Club of West Frankfort, Illinois. Concurrently, Whitaker asked the secretary of each county medical society to get in touch with the personal physicians of members of the state's congressional delegation. The idea was that a congressman would surely pay special attention to a letter from his own doctor. "We will provide form letters," Whitaker promised, "but the society secretary should help the doctor, if necessary, in rewriting and personalizing the letter in each instance."

Dr. Means, among others, took exception to this procedure. "Every doctor is invited to make a political pressure outpost of his private office!" he wrote in the *Atlantic*. "The personal physicians of politicians are being urged to put the heat on these, their patients, to vote right on medical bills. This last seems no longer necessary, as the bills are dead ducks anyway."

46

The suggestion that the A.M.A.'s multimillion-dollar on-slaught amounted to no more than a furious bit of shadow-boxing was not a popular one at A.M.A. headquarters. It was even less popular in the offices of Whitaker & Baxter, since the firm was engaged in a quiet power struggle with Dr. Fishbein over the question of who spoke for the A.M.A. Although Dr. Fishbein had been downgraded since Whitaker's arrival, he had continued to wage his own private war against the government—for the most part, in the pages of the *Journal*. At the A.M.A.'s convention in the summer of 1949, the House of Delegates gave Whitaker & Baxter a standing ovation for the job it was doing and renewed its contract for another year. At the same time, the board of trustees ordered Dr. Fishbein to "completely eliminate speaking on all controversial subjects," and restricted his official duties to working on the *Journal*. "Last June, the American Medical Association withdrew its Seal of Acceptance from Morris Fishbein," Mayer wrote in *Harper's* that fall. "Then, just so there would be no misunderstanding, it beat his head in, cut his heart out, and kicked him into the street. 'If the atmosphere becomes unpleasant,' said the Voice of American Medicine, picking himself up and straightening his necktie, 'I'll quit in five minutes.'" Apparently, an absence of controversy made the atmosphere unpleasant enough, for in December the A.M.A. announced, "regretfully," that Dr. Fishbein had retired, "after thirty-seven years of devoted service."

9

AMID the clamor of the National Education Campaign, another move that organized medicine made in 1949 went largely unnoticed. This was a decision to participate directly in political campaigns. The idea was not a new one. In the mid-thirties, an editorial in the *Journal* of the Indiana State Medical Association had suggested something of the sort:

> Let us inquiringly search out the legislative mesquite and the administrative underbrush and unmistakably brand with blackball votes this coming fall those mavericks whom we have reason to suspect of long-haired theories and pop-eyed reforms as regards goosestepping the medical profession. . . . Otherwise, in their guinea-pig-o-mania, they will march our ideals and idealisms, one by one, up that long, last hill for crucifixion. Once these have been nailed to the cross, then, indeed, it will be too late for us to seek the wailing-wall of remorse. . . . The merely gold-washed chains of ward-healer serfdom await the medical profession if organized medicine slumbers.

Since political activity might have endangered the A.M.A.'s tax-exempt status, opponents of guinea-pig-o-mania had to work independently of the national association. New York was the scene of their first attempt to brand a major candidate of national reputation with a blackball vote. In June, 1949, Senator Wagner resigned from office because of ill-health, and Governor Thomas E. Dewey appointed John Foster Dulles to fill his place until a special election could be held, that November. In mid-September, the Democratic and Liberal Parties chose former Governor Herbert H. Lehman as their candidate, and the Republicans chose Dulles. Although Lehman stated over and over, unequivocally, that he favored voluntary health insurance over compulsory health insurance, doctors around the state were convinced that he was bent on goosestepping the medical profession. A month before the election, a group of them got together and formed a committee called Doctors for Dulles, which was headed by Dr. Charles Gordon Heyd, a past president of both the A.M.A. and the New York State Medical Society. The committee included thirty-five physicians, all either past presidents or former officers of the state society. Their first move was to send letters to more than twenty-six thousand doctors around the state advising them that a vote for Dulles was "a vote against political medicine" and urging them to use their influence "in every possible way" to keep the incumbent in office. Next, Dr. Heyd and his staff met with Governor Dewey and *his* staff to work out a joint strategy. This consisted of dividing the state into twenty-six districts, each with a "healing-arts committee" made up of doctors, dentists, nurses, medical technicians, pharmacists, and people in allied fields. The first order that went out to the "captain" of each committee was: "Familiarize yourself with background of Socialized medicine." That accomplished, the captains were instructed to get the active coöperation of their county medical societies, or, that failing, to "select four or five outstanding doctors in each county who are against Socialized medicine." Each local "working group" was then expected to write a letter to every doctor in the county, followed up by a telephone call, asking him to vote for Dulles. Each doctor was also to be asked to write and telephone everyone he knew with the same request, and to place campaign material in his waiting room—in short, as the instructions urged, "to go all out . . . with his friends and patients."

Nearly eleven thousand physicians in the state coöperated. Before they were through, they had sent more than a million and a quarter letters to patients, had distributed hundreds of thousands of campaign leaflets, had made thousands of telephone calls, and had paid for scores of radio spot announcements and dozens of newspaper advertisements. Dulles lost by two hundred thousand votes, but the doctors who had worked for him drew solace from the belief that their local efforts had helped carry fifty-seven of the state's sixty-two counties for him—that is, all but the five that counted.

The forces of organized medicine were also active in another special election that year, in the Twenty-sixth Congressional District of Pennsylvania. Healing-arts committees there sent out close to two hundred thousand letters to patients and acquaintances, made more than a hundred thousand telephone calls, bought many hours of radio time, and placed advertisements in every newspaper in the district. It was a Republican stronghold, and the Republican candidate, John P. Saylor, who campaigned against national health insurance, won.

At the end of 1949, Whitaker & Baxter, in a report on its activities for the A.M.A., asserted that everything the firm had done had been based on a belief, shared by everyone in the Association, that "the important consideration is not what would happen to doctors under a system of political medicine but what would happen to the American people." That year, the Association reported spending $1,522,683 on lobbying alone, which was the greatest sum ever spent by any lobby—and, in fact, still is. In 1950, organized medicine embarked on an even more elaborate campaign to save the American people from socialized medicine. In February, in a speech before the second national conference of the National Education Campaign, Whitaker recounted the experiences of the healing-arts committees in New York and Pennsylvania, and remarked that there was some talk of setting up similar committees around the country for the forthcoming congressional elections. After reminding his audience that neither the A.M.A. nor its public-relations advisers could legally be associated in any way with these committees, he said, "Without doubt, the most effective single mission doctors can perform in a Congressional campaign, in most districts, is a thoroughgoing letter-writing job, beamed to their patients—*personal* letters, signed by the doctor on his professional letterhead, and mailed in his own envelopes." Within a few months, a surprisingly large number of healing-arts committees had sprung up spontaneously around the country and begun organizing a vast letter-writing campaign.

Although circumscribed by the law, the A.M.A. did have some plans of its own for election time. The previous November, Whitaker, this time in a speech before the National Editorial Association, had told the assembled editors that there was a scurrilous rumor going around, "an absolutely fraudulent story, implying that the managers of the American Medical Association's campaign planned to bribe the American press." Having dismissed the notion as ridiculous, he announced that the A.M.A.'s plans for the following year included a "newspaper advertising schedule," and added, "Every bona fide newspaper in America, every one of the twelve thousand . . . will be in that schedule." In conclusion, he said, "When the time comes that your critics attempt to make the people of this country feel that the press can be bought, and that your editorial columns are for sale; when that propaganda is spread by those in the government or by their agents, I think it is time for American newspapers and American doctors to make common cause and not stop fighting until we throw the rascals out." The advertising schedule that was promised was enormous—probably the greatest in American political history—but Whitaker was as good as his word. In June, the A.M.A.'s board of trustees announced that it had approved an advertising budget of $1,110,000, of which $560,000 would go for large advertisements in every newspaper in the country, $300,000 for radio spot announcements, and $250,000 for magazine advertising. This publicity barrage was to be fired off late in October, just before the elections. "We want the terrific impact of all the media hitting at once," Whitaker explained.

In the meantime, campaign headquarters in Chicago mailed stereotype mats to the advertising directors of more than ten thousand newspapers. Each mat provided space for a tie-in arrangement that could be used by small local concerns, and an accompanying letter pointed out that businesses that ordinarily didn't feel they could afford advertising might be willing to pay for ready-made layouts requiring only the addition of the company's name at the bottom. Thousands of small businessmen went for the idea, including dairy owners ("Selling Milk is Selling Health! . . . Our service to this community has much in common with that of the medical profession"), merchants ("What's Wrong With Freedom? . . . All freedoms stand or fall together. That's why we take our stand today, with the doctors of America, for the Voluntary system"), restaurant, saloon, and soda-fountain proprietors ("There's No Such Thing As a Free Lunch! . . . We want a free America—not the 'free lunch' sort of Government"), and pharmacists ("From Pills to Penicillin . . . This progress is more than statistics—it's people! And the people we know don't want it tampered with!").

Big businesses were by no means ignored. Dr. Elmer Henderson, who was president of the A.M.A. that year, signed a letter that went out to the presidents of twenty-five thousand corporations, urging them to buy tie-in advertising of their own for the big push in October. Before long, representatives of some of the nation's largest insurance companies, railroads, private utilities, pharmaceutical firms, retail chains, and Blue Cross and Blue Shield plans agreed to take their share. "An estimated $19 million will come from these tie-in ads," Jean Begeman reported in the *New Republic*. "Newspaper and radio admen, who have watched this bonanza grow, look to October as the lushest in advertising history." Senator Murray called the bonanza "a tragic waste" and enumerated some of the things that could have been done with the money, such as paying the medical expenses of a hundred and sixty thousand poor families or underwriting the tuition costs of nine thousand medical students—enough to care for six million patients. Instead, the money was paid to carry the A.M.A.'s message in newspapers with a combined circulation of 115,630,487, in magazines with a combined circulation of 55,202,080, and over radio stations with a total of 108,205,-034 listeners. "We didn't have to ask ourselves, at the end of that campaign, where the American people stood," Whitaker said later. "We had dramatic proof of it, not only in the record-breaking amount of tie-in advertising but in the thousands of letters which poured into our offices from all over the nation."

Among a number of developments for which the A.M.A. took credit in 1950 was the defeat of several of its enemies in Congress—Senators Claude Pepper, of Florida, and Frank Graham, of North Carolina, in primary contests, and Senator Elbert Thomas, of Utah, and Representatives Eugene O'Sullivan, of Nebraska, and Andrew Biemiller, of Wisconsin, in the election. Doctors were unquestionably active in these races, but in the opinion of many political analysts at least two of the candidates lost for other reasons—Pepper because he was charged with being soft on Communists, and Graham because he was charged with being soft on Negroes. Whether the number of scalps was three or five, though, it was generally agreed (outside the A.M.A.) that they had been collected at a cost out of all proportion to their value. That year, the A.M.A. reported spending two and a half million dollars on its public-relations campaign and on direct lobbying.

All in all, 1950 was probably the busiest year in the A.M.A.'s history. Even apart from its National Education Campaign, it was unusually active in the capital. Its lobbyists there worked to head off seven health-insurance measures (none of them the Wagner-Murray-Dingell bill, which even its sponsors had given up on) and to block a number of fringe proposals, including bills to expand public-school medical programs; to set up a new department for all health, education, and welfare activities; to give federal aid to various rural health plans, local public-health units, and medical schools; and to provide disability insurance under the Social Security system.

10

UNKNOWN to the A.M.A., some of the forces against which it was waging its war were quietly preparing to open a new front. Ewing, who was under orders from the White House to come up with a health-insurance plan that would be politically acceptable, had been looking around all year for some alternative to the Wagner-Murray-Dingell approach. Finally, near the end of 1950, he and the two aides who had written the Wagner-Murray-Dingell bills, Cohen and Falk, decided to concentrate their efforts on a more or less modest idea that they thought might be put across. As officials of the Federal Security Agency, which ran the Social Security program, they were thoroughly familiar with the problems facing the aged, one of the most burdensome of which was the cost of illness. Although the three men didn't have precise statistics on the matter, they were well aware that older people were far more susceptible to sickness and far less able to pay for medical treatment than any other group. They also knew that hospital costs—the largest item in the medical budget—were rising at a rate of more than five per cent a year, and that the fastest-growing segment of the population consisted of people over sixty-five. Their idea, then, was to provide all men and women who were getting Social Security pensions—some seven million people—with sixty days of free hospital care a year. This approach had been discussed among officials of the Social Security Board as early as 1944, but it had never been taken very seriously, because of the emphasis nearly everyone in those days placed on legislation that would provide much broader coverage.

"Before this, we'd been thinking in the billions," Cohen,

who is now Under Secretary of the Department of Health, Education, and Welfare, recalled recently. "The new idea seemed pretty paltry at first—a trifling two hundred and thirty million dollars a year. In the beginning, we looked at it as a small way of starting something big—what the A.M.A. likes to call 'a foot in the door.' But in time the bill we wrote—or, anyway, the idea behind it—became our *only* goal. Although the doctors are convinced that we intend to expand it downward, to individuals under sixty-five, I don't think a single responsible person in the government has any such intentions. As far as I'm concerned, this is America's form of national health insurance. Anyway, it's all been very Hegelian. The state and federal proposals for compulsory health insurance were the thesis, the A.M.A.'s violent opposition was the antithesis, and Medicare is the synthesis."

In June, 1951, Ewing held a press conference at which he outlined the new plan. "It is difficult for me to see how anyone with a heart can oppose this," he said. Ultimately, the A.M.A. was to oppose it with all its heart, but right then it was too busy lobbying against the moribund Wagner-Murray-Dingell bill, at a cost of almost half a million dollars, to pay much attention to the new proposal. National health insurance in any form seemed to be a dead issue at the time. In his State of the Union Address in 1952, President Truman mentioned it only in general terms. Neither the Democratic platform nor the Party's Presidential candidate that year paid much attention to the issue. On the other hand, General Eisenhower came out firmly against socialized medicine. "I don't like the word 'compulsory,'" he said. In 1952, the A.M.A. spent only a quarter of a million dollars fighting the old Wagner-Murray-Dingell bill, which wasn't introduced in Congress that year. No money was set aside to be used against the Ewing-Cohen-Falk bill to provide medical care for the aged, which was quietly filed that April by Murray in the Senate and by Dingell in the House. "Prospects for action this session appear remote," the *Times* noted afterward.

The A.M.A. apparently believed that the prospects of what has since come to be known as Medicare were nonexistent. In

September, 1952, Dr. Louis H. Bauer, the incumbent president of the Association, announced that the fight against national health insurance had been won, and that the A.M.A.'s National Education Campaign was being disbanded. "The American Medical Association, on this occasion, wishes to thank the American people for their heartening demonstration of confidence and support," Dr. Bauer said. In all, the three-and-a-half-year National Education Campaign for the American people's support had cost the A.M.A. $4,678,000, of which about a third of a million dollars had been Whitaker & Baxter's fee.

Of course, the amount officially spent by the forces of organized medicine represented only part of the total cost. Since federal law does not require that state and local political contributions and expenses be filed, no total can be arrived at with any certainty. However, some idea of it can be derived from one relatively small part of a relatively small campaign —in 1949 the mailing costs of the Doctors for Dulles group came to a hundred and sixty-eight thousand dollars. In addition to expenditures by individual doctors and business allies, which must have run well into the millions during the National Education Campaign, there were certain hidden costs that couldn't be reckoned at the time. For example, one Midwestern congressman with substantial seniority felt that the over-all effect of the floods of mail and petitions he and his colleagues received may have been very different from what the senders intended. "I don't think a man in the House was influenced by that stuff—unless he wanted to use it to justify a position he'd already decided on," he said not long ago. "Most of it was junk—form letters and form resolutions that none of us pay any attention to, because we know they don't represent what our constituents are really thinking. For myself, the A.M.A. blitz had a very strong negative effect. I knew what was in the Wagner-Murray-Dingell bill, and I knew that the A.M.A.'s advertisements and press releases were ridiculous. That kind of campaign, coming from that kind of profession, just disgusted me. Even personally written and obviously sincere letters that I got from some voters in my district who had been misled by this propaganda didn't affect me. I didn't come to Washington to obey the dictates of the misinformed."

Propaganda can be a dangerous weapon to use, and in the country at large the medical profession's immense outlay may have brought about precisely what it least wanted—increased public interest in some form of national health insurance. "Thanks to Whitaker & Baxter, there is a general public awareness that the federal government *could* do something about the health of the nation," an editorial in the magazine *Survey* pointed out at the time. "Eventually, organized medicine may discover it has rendered a public service it never intended paying for."

11

AMONG the many tactical games played on Capitol Hill, one of the favorites is known informally as "building a record"—a record for or against a given piece of legislation. Although members of Congress and their aides often play it with impressive skill, endurance, and ferocity, it is not much of a spectator sport. The information that staff researchers collect, or are given, to support their case usually consists of charts, graphs, tables of statistics, and other cumbersomely undramatic material. Once arranged in some kind of order, it is introduced in committee hearings, which few people attend, and then winnowed out of the printed transcript and presented in the committee's majority or minority report, which few people read—mainly because the only people who are really interested in it had a hand in putting it together in the first place. Another approach is for a senator or a representative to rise on the floor while Congress is in session and make a speech that adds to the record—in this case, the *Congressional Record*. While this technique doesn't call for the virtuosity that is sometimes required in the courtroom atmosphere of a hearing, it does call for an unusual ability to suspend any sense of the absurd on the part of the speaker, who, far more often than not, will find himself speaking to an almost empty chamber; this is especially hard on the old-fashioned orators who roar and wave their arms and pound their desks as a colleague or two nods sleepily or reads the paper, and tourists in the gallery watch in bewilderment. On the other hand, the method has certain advantages. If a member makes a mistake or is questioned to his detriment by an opponent who happens to wander in, he is allowed, under the rules of the game, to edit his comments before the *Record* goes to press; of course, this causes some confusion when the questioner fails to alter his remarks, too, but no one seems to mind. To be even safer, a member can send over a prepared speech and not appear at all. Although he may actually be lolling on the beach at Montego Bay, as far as the *Record* and history are concerned it will appear that he was in the thick of it. In any event, the game itself often seems to be more important than the final score. When things don't come off as planned during a hearing, or a bill fails to get voted out of committee, or a subject is temporarily set aside by an adversary's parliamentary maneuver, or a bill is defeated in a floor vote, the remark made by the supporters of a particular measure is invariably something like "Well, we lost that round, but we got a lot of good stuff in the record." With that excuse, hundreds of acres of Canadian forest are depleted each year. And, by and large, the printed records they are used for accomplish little except to reduce the available space in the Archives. Even so, the game has to be played out, because no bill of any consequence is approved by Congress until it has been buttressed by enough evidence to justify its passage in the minds of those who must do the voting.

In this century, by far the most extensive game of building a record—one that wore out several teams on both sides—revolved around the issue of government health insurance. Although by 1952 the A.M.A. was boasting that it had won the game, once and for all, actually the contest was just beginning. Between 1912 and 1952, according to a government researcher who helped compile statistics on the medical needs of the population as a whole, several trainloads of data must have been collected, collated, and published. Now these were shunted off onto a siding as the government began to concentrate on studying medical care—or the lack of it—for the elderly. The first major submission to the new record was made toward the end of 1952. In December of the previous year, President Truman had set up a Commission on the Health Needs of the Nation, consisting of a group of prominent citizens in medicine, public health, education, and labor, who were instructed to make a study and to turn in their findings to him within a year.

Under the direction of Dr. Paul Magnuson—who was a noted surgeon, a Republican, and an outspoken opponent of national health insurance—the commission held extensive hearings around the country, and then submitted its report to Mr. Truman a few weeks before he left office. The report delighted some people, including the President; it infuriated others, including the A.M.A.; and it surprised everyone else, since the appointment of the commission had generally been looked upon as the administration's way of conceding that any action on federal health insurance was, just as the A.M.A. had claimed, highly unlikely. The commission's report stated that "access to the means for attainment and preservation of health is a basic human right"—a right so many Americans were being deprived of, it continued, that the government would be justified in spending a billion dollars a year on additional care for the people's health.

While the report covered just about every kind of medical problem, it devoted an unexpected amount of attention to the health needs of the elderly. "It is clear that the solution to the problem of payment for health services to the aging does not lie in currently available private insurance programs with premiums paid by the aging," the report stated. Then it went on to say, "Rather, the situation requires a new approach— one supported largely by public funds specifically earmarked for health care." In conclusion, it recommended that "funds collected through the Old-Age and Survivors Insurance mechanism [the Social Security program] be utilized to purchase personal health service benefits on a pre-payment basis for beneficiaries of that insurance program, under a plan which meets federal standards and which does not involve a means test."

Dr. Bauer, president of the A.M.A., condemned the commission's recommendation at once, saying that the proposal had already been "rejected repeatedly by the American people," and that the report contained "numerous false and contradictory conclusions." If the *Times* was correct in an observation it made later—that "the A.M.A. is the sworn enemy of whatever . . . threatens to tamper with the doctor's immemorial right to charge whatever he believes the traffic will bear"—the A.M.A. had reason to be concerned about some of the implications of the recommendation. Ultimately, just about everyone agreed, "federal standards" would mean some measure of federal control, and when the government was footing the bill, it would sooner or later take a look at what it was paying for. Furthermore, the absence of a means test—that is, a test to prove that an applicant for welfare is too poor to care for himself—might well lead to the establishment of a standard fee for patients who could pay as well as for patients who couldn't, and, in all likelihood, would bring that fee down from what the traffic would bear to what the federal government would bear.

The means test, which the A.M.A. fought for to the end, was at the heart of the ensuing controversy. A program that provided medical care only for those who were unable to pay for it at the market price made that care charity. On the other hand, a program that provided medical care for Social Security beneficiaries under an insurance system that they had contributed to made that care an earned right. The means test, an offspring of the Elizabethan poor laws, has long been almost unanimously condemned by welfare experts as a cruel indignity visited on people who, through no fault of their own, have little enough self-respect to begin with. (Not long ago, it was more than an indignity; as late as the mid-thirties, fourteen states considered success in a means test sufficient cause to deprive a welfare recipient of the right to vote.)

The means test has also been a psychological obstacle to the acceptance of assistance by those who are old, sick, and poor. According to Edward T. Chase, a writer on the social aspects of medicine, "the empirical evidence shows that the means test has acted to prevent needed medical care for an untold number of the elderly infirm by discouraging them from applying for assistance." In many jurisdictions, means tests include what is called "relative responsibility"—that is, the responsibility of relatives (including in-laws) to exhaust

61

their own assets before welfare help is given. Under this system, banks are circularized for evidence of holdings, and any assets such as homes, personal belongings, life-insurance, and burial-insurance policies have to be disposed of and the money used up before assistance is given.

On the statistical side, the President's commission added a large amount of significant data to the record. To begin with, the report revealed, since 1900 the number of people sixty-five years old and over had risen from three million to twelve and a half million, and from four per cent of the total population to eight per cent. At the same time, people over sixty-five were hospitalized twice as long and were incapacitated by chronic illnesses five times as often as those under sixty-five. And while hospital costs were rising at a steady rate of between five and seven per cent a year, some two-thirds of the aged had incomes of less than a thousand dollars a year. Only one in eight elderly couples had any kind of health insurance, the report continued, and explained, "They are considered 'bad' risks by insurance organizations and even if eligible the premiums would usually be beyond their means." Moreover, people in this country were not only living longer but retiring earlier, with the result that both their incomes and their savings were lower. The elderly, who were almost as numerous as the total of the unemployed during the Depression, often lived under conditions that were reminiscent of that period.

One witness who testified at the commission's hearings in Dallas—Dr. George W. Jackson, Medical Director of the Board for Texas State Hospitals and Special Schools—described some of the changes that had taken place in the lives of the aged over the past generation or so:

In the early days when most of the people lived on farms in rural settings with large homes and plenty of individualized work, the aged in our population could be housed and cared for without interfering with the over-all activity of the family group. There were jobs for everyone to do, and these jobs varied in the amount of physical and mental effort necessary to effect them. In this situation there was work for all but the most severely handicapped persons. Added to this was the fact that families were large and there were always hands available to help handle and feed the disabled or infirm.

This picture has entirely changed in the past fifty years, for now instead of the farm with its large family group, we have the modern efficiency apartment or small home with its one- or two-child family. Few, if any, jobs are available in or around the modern homestead. . . . In this new situation there is no work adaptable for the old and the infirm, and there are no friendly hands to guide and feed them in time of need.

Dr. Jackson went on to point out that, despite the Social Security program, the rising cost of living and the reduced span of working years made it next to impossible for most people to accumulate enough savings by retirement age for anything but the bare necessities, and in many cases not even enough for those. Of every hundred men who were twenty-five years old in 1952, he said, sixty-five would live to the age of retirement; of these, one would have above-average means, nine would be able to scrape by, and the fifty-five others would become public charges. The report itself forecast that there would be twenty million people sixty-five years old and older in the United States by 1970, and that most of them would be unable to feed, clothe, and house themselves adequately, let alone pay the doctor.

12

A PROBLEM that affects many millions of people cannot be ignored indefinitely in a political system like ours. "When the Eisenhower people took over in 1953, they didn't seem to realize the immense political potential of this group," Wilbur Cohen, the co-author of the 1952 bill, recalled not long ago. "At the time, there were between twelve and thirteen million people over sixty-five, and every day there were a thousand more, almost all of whom were eligible to vote, and most of whom did. That's a massive political bloc. Generally speaking, older people are conservatives, but not when it comes to Social Security increases or government participation in health care. During the Eisenhower administration, I conducted a survey that showed they were strongly in favor of federal health insurance. Anyway, our bill was extremely limited, compared to earlier and later proposals. It provided for a small increase in Social Security premiums so that people could pay during their working years into a fund that would later give them a couple of months of hospital care, which is the largest single expense in the medical budget. If the A.M.A. had supported the plan, the doctors could have got control of it, and the whole business would have stopped there. But they weren't willing to accept anything at all. And neither was the Eisenhower administration."

The A.M.A.'s opposition was based on a conviction that national health insurance for a limited group would inevitably lead to national health insurance for everyone. President Eisenhower's opposition was said to be related to commitments he had made in exchange for support from organized medicine and the insurance industry during the 1952 campaign. At any rate, it is known that shortly after taking office he assured the A.M.A. that the government would stay out of medical affairs if the A.M.A. would not oppose the creation of a new Cabinet post to coördinate the government's health, education, and welfare activities. President Truman had tried to set up this post for years, but the A.M.A. had opposed him at every turn.

When General Eisenhower also promised the A.M.A. that it could choose the department's special assistant for medical affairs, the A.M.A. relented, and in the spring of 1953 the department known in Washington as H.E.W. came into being. Its first Secretary, Mrs. Oveta Culp Hobby, announced that her stewardship would be "an A.M.A. administration." According to a man who worked for her, she did her best to keep her promise. "But the doctors that the Association recommended for the post of special assistant were so, let us say, unremarkable that not even Mrs. Hobby would accept them," he recalled recently. "The word we got was that none of their really qualified men would work for a government salary." Finally, H.E.W. was forced to turn to the academic world for a first-rate man—Dr. Lowell T. Coggleshell, dean of the division of biological sciences at the University of Chicago. As it happened, he was a liberal and not acceptable to the A.M.A., but since the Association was unable to come up with a man of its own, there was little it could do now. The intimacy between the White House and the A.M.A. was briefly shaken later that year when President Eisenhower, having heard that the Association was claiming to have been solely responsible for his election, sent word through an intermediary that he did not look kindly on statements of this sort.

In 1953, Senator Murray and Representative Dingell again introduced their bill, although there seemed to be no hope of getting it out of committee now that the Republicans who had been swept into office along with Eisenhower were in control of Congress. No hearings were held on the bill, but its very existence and the stir caused by the commission's report unsettled the A.M.A., and Mrs. Hobby came up with a plan that she felt would satisfy everybody. (She came up with it one hour after Falk, the co-author of the Murray-Dingell bill, had left her department to return to private life.) Her proposal—called government reinsurance—was to provide an annual federal subsidy of twenty-five million dollars to be spread out among private insurance companies that would take on the risk of writing low-cost health-insurance policies. The bill was submitted to Congress and sent to the Senate Committee on Labor and Public Welfare, which duly reported it out and passed it on to the Senate for a vote.

A dissenting member of a committee usually expresses his views in a statement at the end of the committee's majority report. In this case, Senator Murray, who had been chairman of the committee until the Republicans took over, issued a separate report, in which he attacked the bill as "a paltry, puny, picayune proposal." Then he went on in a way that variously amused, pained, and shocked his colleagues:

It is not too surprising that individual members of the present administration seem not to understand the problem or to have any idea as to what to do about it. After all, President Eisenhower cannot be held responsible for a lack of acquaintance with this field. For all his adult life he has not only been completely out of touch with the economic problems besetting the average American family but, as regards the problem of a family's paying for medical care, he has simply never been confronted with it. Like members of the Congress, the President has had available a most complete medical-care service, provided, without charge, by the American taxpayer through physicians and dentists working for the government on salary. In short, since President Eisenhower has been getting free, socialized medical care almost all his adult life, it is obvious that there is no reason why he personally would have developed any real understanding of this particular problem. . . . In attempting to explain to myself just why the administration should have devised and offered us so strange a proposal, I have found one conclusion inescapable. . . . It was intended to lead the American people into believing that the administration was seriously concerned and was really doing something about the impossible costs of medical care, while at the same time it would lull into a sense of security those

66

who had contributed so much time, effort, and money to the Republican campaign of 1952 because they believed that a vested interest in the established system of paying for medical care would be protected.

Murray's attack, along with the fact that no one except Mrs. Hobby was enthusiastic about the bill, defeated it then and there in the Senate. Minority Leader Sam Rayburn, who was angry at Mrs. Hobby, a Democrat and a Texan, for accepting a Cabinet post in a Republican administration, saw to it that the bill was defeated over in the House.

When the Eighty-fourth Congress convened in 1955, the Murray-Dingell bill was again introduced, and again it got nowhere. An event of far greater significance that year was the merger of two groups that had always been the largest, most active, and most powerful supporters of national health insurance—the American Federation of Labor and the Congress of Industrial Organizations, which together represented more than sixteen million workers. But before tackling health insurance the new labor giant tested its strength on a less important piece of legislation that unions had wanted for a long time—payment of Social Security benefits to those past the age of fifty who were totally disabled. The chief antagonist in this contest, too, was the A.M.A., which contended, primarily, that the proposal would give the government authority to determine a person's medical condition, that it would cost too much, and that it would encourage malingering.

According to many critics of the A.M.A., its Whitaker & Baxter "educational" campaigns back in the nineteen-forties and early fifties had done serious damage to one of the Association's greatest assets—its standing as an objective scientific organization. When the disability bill came up, it was reported that the A.M.A. had turned to another public-relations outfit, and that this one had devised a far more strident campaign than anything Whitaker & Baxter had come up with. Finally, some friends in Congress prevailed on the Association to proceed with caution this time, and even an A.M.A. official later conceded that the advice had merit. "We would have looked awful," he said. "Can you imagine going to the public and seeming to argue that it's subversive to give Social Security to a disabled workman? We'd have been tarred and feathered as being against cripples." In the end, the A.M.A.'s lobbyists did their work in the old-fashioned way—along the corridors and in the offices and cloakrooms on Capitol Hill. The fight was a bitter and protracted one, but the A.F.L.-C.I.O. ultimately won it, and the bill was enacted in 1956. (The program cost so little and was so successful that Congress later removed the age limit.)

As an innovation, the new law was fairly insignificant, but as a precedent it was substantial. That same year, the A.M.A. failed to stop the expansion of another legislative precedent. Back in 1950, Congress had passed a modest bill, over A.M.A. opposition, giving the federal government the authority to provide very small matching grants to the states, under the Old Age Assistance program, for "medical-vender" payments —that is, payments to doctors and others providing medical care. This meant that for the first time the federal government was making payments to provide medical services instead of merely giving out cash to be used as the recipient saw fit. In 1956, Congress enlarged this program considerably by making more funds available to the states. The A.M.A. was apparently so preoccupied with the disability fight that it failed to realize that this move presented a far graver threat than the disability bill. In any event, the Association did nothing more than write a letter expressing its disapproval to the committee that was considering the "medical-vender" proposal. Members of Congress, who were accustomed to more pressure than that on anything the A.M.A. cared about, concluded that the doctors didn't really object, and quickly passed the measure.

While precedents are often crucial in the business of interpreting laws, they are usually important in the business of making laws only when the public is demanding action anyway and lawmakers decide to use them. Of far greater consequence than any number of precedents like the disability and vender-payment legislation of 1956 could have been, in the long run, was an idea that William Reidy, a member of the staff of the Senate Committee on Labor and Public Welfare, passed on indirectly, early that year, to Senator John F. Kennedy, who was a low-ranking member of the committee. In discussions with other staff members, Reidy had become convinced that the problems of the increasing number of older people in this country were acute and that they affected far more people than just the elderly themselves—mainly their children, who often had to support or otherwise take care of them, but also their grandchildren, and even their great-grandchildren, who were likely to be deprived of educational advantages when a family's savings were used to pay for the care of aged relatives.

Believing that these circumstances indicated a growing social crisis, and thus an imminent political issue, Reidy decided that the time had come to set up a new Senate subcommittee on the aging. The next step was to find a senator who would take up the cause—preferably a senator with high ambitions and little national exposure. Like most people working on the Hill, Reidy had heard that Senator Kennedy had his eye on the White House and thus might be favorably disposed toward a proposal that could make him widely known outside his home state. When Reidy went to Kennedy's office to present his case, he got as far as Theodore Sorensen, then, as later, Kennedy's closest associate. Sorensen heard Reidy out, shook his head, and dismissed the subject with the assertion that Senator Kennedy would never be interested in the problems of the elderly. Unwilling to leave it at that, Reidy later managed to pass his idea on to the senator through another associate, and it turned out that Kennedy was very much interested. He was too busy just then with a subcommittee of his own—the Subcommittee on Labor—to take on a new one.

Not long afterward, though, he found time to co-sponsor, with Senator Lister Hill, of Alabama, the chairman of his parent committee, an omnibus bill dealing with all the problems of the elderly that they could think of. Known as the Senior Citizens Opportunity and Security bill, it had been drafted by Wilbur Cohen, who had left H.E.W. to become a professor of public welfare administration at the University of Michigan, and who was Kennedy's adviser on Social Security matters. Hill and Kennedy introduced the measure in the Senate late that June, but there was little interest in it, and it never came to a vote. However, it had one indirect result that summer: the Senate passed a resolution, introduced by Hill, to appropriate thirty thousand dollars for a study of the aged and aging, which Reidy hoped would ultimately lead to the appointment of a subcommittee on the subject. Under Cohen's direction, a ten-volume report was compiled at the Library of Congress. Nothing came of that, either—except, of course, that it was added to the record.

13

THE Constitution gives Congress "all legislative powers herein granted" and gives the President the right to "recommend . . . such measures as he shall judge necessary and expedient," but it says nothing about where legislation may or must be conceived. Most of it is conceived in the offices of lobbyists. To many people this seems possibly illegal, probably unethical, and certainly a perversion of the democratic process. It is none of these. Under the First Amendment, the people are expressly granted the right "to petition the government for a redress of grievances," and there is surely no more cogent petition than a precisely drafted bill. Moreover, of the hundreds of pieces of legislation that are written each year in lobbyists' offices a fair number are written at the request of members of Congress. There are several reasons for such requests. One is that a member of Congress rarely has the staff to do this sort of work himself; another is that he is seldom as expert on a subject as a man who has made it his specialty; and a third is that if he hopes to get his bill passed, he might as well line up the support of special-interest groups right at the beginning. This is not to say that the legislators invariably sell out to the lobbyists. While most of the major bills affecting business, farm, and labor groups are apt to be originally drafted by the national organizations representing those special interests, the drafts are generally rewritten by members of Congress to fit their special needs—or, on occasion, to serve the public interest.

Late in 1956, the A.F.L.-C.I.O., which has produced its share of bills over the years, decided to step up the gradual movement toward some form of health insurance for the elderly. Nelson Cruikshank, a former Methodist minister who had become director of the A.F.L.-C.I.O.'s Department of Social Security, got together with Robert Ball, one of the top men in the United States Social Security Administration, and with the two men who had drafted the 1952 Murray-Dingell bill— Cohen and his former H.E.W. colleague, I. S. Falk. Before long, the four men, conferring largely by telephone and letter, had prepared a new and greatly expanded bill to provide medical care for Social Security beneficiaries.

Like its predecessor, the bill gave the elderly sixty days of hospitalization, but it went on to cover the costs of surgery and of care in nursing homes. Hospitals, doctors, and nursing homes were free to join the plan or stay out of it, and patients were free to choose any of the physicians or institutions participating. In addition, it was made clear that "nothing in the provisions of the bill . . . shall be construed to give the Secretary of Health, Education, and Welfare [who was to administer the program] supervision or control over, first, the practice of medicine or the manner in which medical services are provided; second, the details of administration or operation of hospitals or nursing homes; or, third, the selection, tenure, or compensation of hospital or nursing-home personnel." The benefits were to be paid for by increasing the amount of income on which Social Security taxes were levied from $4,200 to $6,000 (enough to allow a sweetener in the form of a ten-per-cent increase in payments to everyone covered by Social Security) and by increasing the tax rate itself by one-half of one per cent for both employees and employers. These changes, an H.E.W. actuary reported, would produce enough revenue to pay for the annual cost of the bill—around eight hundred million dollars.

At this point, Cruikshank called in Andrew Biemiller, the A.F.L.-C.I.O.'s Director of Legislation—that is, its chief lobbyist—because the time had now arrived for an approach to Congress. It was an approach that Biemiller, a former congressman from Wisconsin, was happy to make, for back in 1950 doctors in Wisconsin had put on a high-powered political campaign that he thought had played a part in defeating him for reëlection. The seniority system on Capitol Hill is respected not only by members of Congress but by individuals and groups who want something from them, so Biemiller and Cruikshank, looking for a sponsor, took the bill to the chairman of the House Committee on Ways and Means, which is responsible for all tax legislation. The Democrats had regained control of Congress in the 1954 elections, and the committee's chairman was Representative Jere Cooper, of Tennessee. Cooper, who was ill and was also occupied with other legislative concerns, turned the two men down, and so, in short order, did the second man in line on the committee's Democratic majority, Wilbur Mills, of Arkansas, and the third man, Noble Gregory, of Kentucky.

Biemiller and Cruikshank had expected this kind of reception, for organized labor wasn't a big factor in any of these men's districts, so they trudged on to the fourth man in line— Aimé Forand, of Rhode Island. Forand wasn't enthusiastic about the idea, but he didn't reject it out of hand. Seizing on his hesitation, the two men plugged away, with descriptions of the bill's merits and all sorts of assurances to ease his misgivings. Finally, and somewhat reluctantly, Forand gave in, and on August 27th, just a few days before the 1957 session adjourned, he rose in the House chamber and submitted the bill. Although Forand told his colleagues at the time that he hoped for action on the bill the following year, he admitted privately that he didn't expect anything to come of it for ten years or more. Not long afterward, however, Selig Greenberg, a reporter for the Providence *Journal* who was friendly with some influential men in the A.F.L.-C.I.O., began writing articles for his paper about the great enthusiasm for the bill that was being displayed by elderly citizens in Rhode Island. Before long, Forand had become far more interested in the measure and far more optimistic about its prospects.

Over the years, the A.M.A. had become convinced that the one great danger it faced was the government's determination to pass a bill that would make health insurance compulsory for every man, woman, and child in the nation. Because of its obsession with this notion—what one doctor later called a

"Maginot Line complex"—it didn't appear to be aware that the Forand bill might sweep clear around its defenses. In 1957, the A.M.A. spent only fifty thousand dollars on lobbying, compared to a million and a half dollars in the peak year of 1949. By the end of 1957, it had finally noticed the flank attack, but still wasn't paying much attention to it. That December, at a meeting of the House of Delegates, the president of the Association described the new bill as "at least nine parts evil and one part sincerity."

Apparently the evil parts didn't look too threatening at the time. It wasn't until the following spring that the A.M.A. took action—by setting up a Joint Council to Improve the Health Care of the Aged, which was to be made up of the A.M.A., the American Hospital Association, the American Dental Association, and the American Nursing Home Association. The title turned out to be a misnomer, for the council's chief conclusion was that the health care of the aged didn't need improving. Not only were the aged getting top-notch medical care, it reported, but they were far better off economically and in most other respects than younger people were. Indeed, the council urged everyone to consider not the problems of the elderly but their opportunities. One congressman who had not taken a position on the Forand bill at the time later said that the council's statements convinced him that the elderly must be in terrible shape. "It was the approach that made me suspicious," he said. "You know, when a large bread producer, say, starts talking in its advertisements about all its busy little bakers and their old-fashioned methods, you can be pretty sure the place has just been automated."

At the time, critics of the A.M.A. claimed that the council was nothing but a public-relations gimmick, its purposes being to enlist new allies in the fight against the Forand bill and to demonstrate a formidable united front against the bill by those who were most closely involved with medical care. If the council did have these purposes, it must have been a considerable source of disappointment to the A.M.A. Shortly after it was formed, some people began asking why its participants didn't include the American Nurses' Association, which had a hundred and seventy thousand members. A couple of months later, the question was answered when the nurses announced that they endorsed the principle behind the Forand bill and might well endorse the bill itself before long. Just after that happened, the American Hospital Association, despite its participation in the council, stated that something along the lines of the Forand proposal might "be necessary ultimately."

It was clear that while the advocates of limited government health insurance were gaining in strength and determination, its opponents were losing some of theirs. Throughout the nineteen-thirties and early forties, organized medicine had successfully maintained discipline in its ranks—chiefly by actual or implied threats of reprisal against dissenters, by scare slogans about the perils of socialized medicine, and by word-of-mouth warnings about what government interference would do to physicians' incomes. But shortly after the Second World War, the development of new and highly complex medical technology and the rapid expansion of health facilities had begun to weaken the A.M.A.'s control. Starting in 1947, the government's annual grants for medical research (initially opposed by the A.M.A.) increased rapidly from twenty-seven million dollars until by 1958 they had reached almost a third of a billion dollars. And it was in 1946 that Congress passed the Hill-Burton bill, which provided federal grants to build, remodel and expand hospitals around the country.

Although the A.M.A. has credited the astonishing progress made in medicine in the past couple of decades to the special virtues of private practice on a fee basis, or what it calls "free-enterprise medicine," most of the progress was actually subsidized by public money—first for research and then for new and expanded hospitals in which the new diagnostic, surgical, and therapeutic techniques developed by research could be put into practice. Formerly, the bulk of medical practice had been conducted in the patient's home and the doctor's office. Now it moved into the hospital, and with it moved a good part of organized medicine's power. Then, too, the doctor in academic life, who had long been suspicious of the A.M.A., gained in stature during this period, for he had developed many of the new techniques, and his views were dominant in the best hospitals—that is, the hospitals with medical-school affiliations.

At the same time, as medicine became a far more exact and efficacious science than ever before, it became far more expensive for those who needed it. To many experts in the fields of medicine, economics, and sociology, it became increasingly clear that the only way of spreading the cost burden around was to adopt some form of health insurance. By the end of the nineteen-forties, labor leaders had begun to concentrate on getting private health-insurance coverage for their members through collective bargaining with employers—and were having far more success than anyone had anticipated. This shift not only led to a remarkable growth in commercial and non-profit health-insurance plans, thus further diluting the A.M.A.'s influence in the health field, but also provided an abundance of statistics on the costs of medical care to enrich the record.

Still another development that weakened the A.M.A.'s once united front was the growing number of physicians working on salary in industry, in government, in universities, in hospitals, in private foundations, and elsewhere. Within less than a generation, the proportion of salaried doctors had risen from ten per cent to more than twenty-five per cent. These physicians—there were some sixty thousand of them in the late nineteen-fifties—were generally independent of A.M.A. control, and they had little or no personal stake in any argument over the sanctity of fees. Finally, the proliferation of specialties and subspecialties led to a corresponding proliferation of specialty societies, and these still further diluted the A.M.A.'s power.

14

ON June 16, 1958, the House Ways and Means Committee, under the direction of its new chairman, Representative Mills, who took over after Congressman Cooper died in 1957, opened hearings on the Forand bill. The lead-off witness was Marion B. Folsom, Mrs. Hobby's successor at H.E.W. To no one's surprise, he testified that the Eisenhower administration opposed the bill. (To many people's surprise, it was later divulged that Folsom privately favored the bill, although he was obliged to oppose it publicly.) The reason for the administration's opposition, he explained, could be found in the phenomenal growth of voluntary health insurance. Between 1952 and 1958, he said, the number of people covered by hospitalization policies had risen from ninety-one million to a hundred and twenty-one million; the number covered by surgical-insurance policies had risen from seventy-three million to a hundred and nine million; and the number covered by general medical-insurance policies had risen from thirty-six million to seventy-two million. Because of this astonishing development in the private sector of the economy, Folsom said, it was the administration's view that the government should not interfere.

The Secretary's position was endorsed by many other witnesses, among them some spokesmen for the insurance industry, which opposed both the health insurance and the Social Security increase provided for in the Forand bill, on the ground that they would cut into the sale of insurance. During both the First and Second World Wars, the insurance industry had opposed government life insurance for servicemen, and had also opposed every increase in Social Security benefits—on the same ground. In the opinion of many economists, the prodigious increase in commercial life and retirement insurance was chiefly due to these government programs, which had not only created an interest in the value of insurance but had released money so that more people could buy it. Now E. J. Faulkner, the spokesman for the Health Insurance Association of America, which represented two hundred and sixty-four companies, avoided taking the usual position and argued instead that the cost of the Forand bill—not, he said, $835,000,000 a year, as its proponents predicted, but $2,112,600,000—would put the entire Social Security program in actuarial jeopardy. In any case, he added, elderly people were already well taken care of under private insurance plans.

On the question of costs, the Eisenhower administration's own figures indicated that the bill would cost less than a billion dollars a year and that there was no danger of its unbalancing the Social Security budget. As for how well off the elderly were under existing conditions, Cruikshank, appearing for the A.F.L.-C.I.O., cited a survey conducted by the United States Public Health Service in 1956, which indicated that a great many people over sixty-five were not getting much benefit out of the phenomenal growth of voluntary health insurance. "Nearly six million of the aged were living in families whose total incomes were under three thousand dollars, and seven out of ten of these aged persons had no health-insurance protection whatever," he said. "Of the two and four-tenths million aged persons not in families, half had incomes under one thousand dollars, and only one-fifth of this half had any health insurance." Moreover, he testified, the majority of the policies held by older people covered only a small proportion of their medical costs, and more than one company cancelled an elderly holder's policy after his first illness. (In fact, a company sometimes cut it off in the middle of an illness, by simply refusing to renew it when a premium payment fell due.) "We have letter after letter in our files . . . [from] people who carry their insurance and pay their premiums for years and then, after the first spell of illness, after retirement age, the company cancels out," Cruikshank said.

Another study he brought up, this one made by the Superintendent of Insurance of New York State, showed that even in those voluntary health-insurance plans that provided the broadest and fullest coverage—group programs under joint industry and union sponsorship—only thirty per cent of the participants were covered after retirement, and most of those who *were* covered had been obliged to convert their old policies to new ones, usually with very high premiums. Of course, for the almost ten million people over sixty-five who had incomes of less than a thousand dollars a year any cost was likely to be prohibitive. And for the million and a half of these who had medical bills averaging seven hundred dollars a year any cost was out of the question. As the study went on to show, elderly people with individual policies were far worse off than elderly people with group policies. Of the million and a half men and women of all ages surveyed in the New York study eighty per cent of those who were insured by individual policies had policies that were cancellable after the first claim and nineteen per cent had policies that were noncancellable only up to a certain age—usually sixty. "Only one per cent had protection as permanent and assured as would result from the Forand bill," Cruikshank concluded.

By far the best insurance plans, it appeared from the testimony, were the ones originally offered by Blue Cross and Blue Shield. But these groups, even though they were non-profit ventures, were hard pressed to go on providing adequate coverage for the elderly. For some years after the two plans got under way, in the thirties, they offered fairly comprehensive coverage at low premiums, but as the members got older and became poorer risks, the premiums had to be raised for everyone participating in order to cover the additional costs. Commercial insurance companies that set up similar programs for businesses stuck to younger workers, and so were able to compete, premium for premium and benefit for benefit, with Blue Cross and Blue Shield. As a result, the commercial plans siphoned off more and more of the better risks, leaving the sick and the elderly to the non-profit plans. (By the end of 1958, these circumstances had driven Blue Cross forty million dollars into the red.) In many states, Blue Cross and Blue Shield took what seemed to be the only way out: they both raised rates and restricted benefits for the elderly. From this standpoint, the aged were worse off, rather than better off, as a result of the growth of voluntary health insurance. As the *Reporter* observed about that time, "From the actuarial standpoint, most of the aged are simply not insurable on a profit basis or even on a break-even basis."

Although the record that was gradually being built up was expressed largely in rather dry statistical terms, the statistics drew more and more serious attention in Washington and elsewhere to the desperate conditions in which millions of old people were living. It was revealed, for example, that one of every four beds in public mental hospitals was occupied by a patient over the age of sixty-five, and that in the opinion of many geriatricians a disturbing number of these elderly patients in mental hospitals were suffering from premature senility induced by a fear of illness and a sense of economic helplessness. In the entire population, it was estimated, half the people with incomes under a thousand dollars a year had illnesses that were not being treated, while only a tenth of the people with incomes over five thousand dollars a year were in that situation.

The attitudes of old people who were too poor to pay for regular medical attention and too proud to go to a charity ward—or, perhaps, too ashamed to force their relatives to undergo a financial investigation—were described by an official spokesman of the Community Council of Greater New York, who said, in part, "The elderly in particular cling fiercely to their waning independence on near-starvation incomes and refuse to apply for public assistance. Others with painful disabilities climb four-flight walkups in preference to moving in with a married child or entering a home for the aged." Of course, there were no statistics available on the number of old people whose near-starvation incomes had driven them to

80

scavenge for food in street-corner wastebaskets, or to pick up rotting fruits and vegetables early in the morning outside produce markets. But the members of the Ways and Means Committee *were* told that many of the old people living on the fringes of American society lacked adequate food as well as adequate medical care. They were also told—repeatedly—that the United States stood eleventh in the world in terms of its citizens' longevity—after Norway, Sweden, Denmark, the Netherlands, West Germany, Iceland, Canada, Israel, Cyprus, and Japan, all of which had some form of government health insurance.

In rebuttal, Dr. Leonard Larson, chairman of the board of the A.M.A., testified that the Forand bill would create a "tremendous and unpredictable drain on the Social Security trust fund," and that it would "legislate the aged into a permanent state of dependency." Representative Forand was more interested in another A.M.A. charge—that his bill amounted to socialized medicine—and he asked Dr. Larson for a definition of the term. This exchange followed:

Dr. LARSON: Mr. Forand, I think it is very difficult to define "socialized medicine." I know of nothing in the record of our Association that would spell out what the Association thinks is socialized medicine.

Mr. FORAND: Dr. Allman [president of the A.M.A.] labelled my bill "socialized medicine." I would like to know just what you mean by "socialized medicine."

Dr. LARSON: He was speaking as the president of the American Medical Association and as an individual, sir.

All in all, the A.M.A. made little attempt to challenge the record that had been built up so far. Dr. Larson was at the witness table for less than half an hour, and none of the other A.M.A. witnesses did much more than ask the committee to accept the A.M.A. view of the bill. "They were invited to appear as expert witnesses, but they displayed no expertise at all," one member of the committee later remarked. "I know that I didn't care for their presentation, and a number of my colleagues didn't, either. We knew there was something in the air—those millions of old people stirring out in our districts—

and some of us were sure that sooner or later a bill like this was inevitable. And the members of the committee who didn't like the bill—by far the majority at the time—were looking to the A.M.A. for some help, some way to defend their position back home. I'm afraid they didn't get anything except the usual hokum."

Much of the material submitted for the record by the A.M.A.'s state societies and individual members was in the form of threats to disobey the law if it was passed and of obvious distortions. Among the dozens of documents filed were a resolution adopted by the Texas Medical Association forbidding its officers to "enter into any contracts or renew any existing contracts which make a governmental organization and the Texas Medical Association parties thereto when the purpose of such contract is the offering of medical care to any group of citizens;" a claim by the Missouri State Medical Association that the bill "would place a tremendous burden on the working public," since "it would hike their taxes for Social Security more than seventy per cent;" a letter from a doctor in Ohio complaining that the measure "would destroy the self-respect of our elderly people;" a letter from a doctor in California stating that his son believed the world owed him a living, and adding his own belief that "something for nothing has already gone too far;" and a speech by an officer of the Association of American Physicians and Surgeons, an ultra right-wing group whose fifteen thousand members were also members of the A.M.A., telling his associates that "this bill, if passed, will be such a strong endorsement of the philosophy of Social Security, and will fix so firmly upon the American people the shackles of the welfare state, that most of you here in this room will live to see the total and permanent destruction of individual freedom."

15

UNLESS a member of Congress wants to indulge in a bit of political grandstanding, he will, at all costs, avoid an adverse vote on a measure he has sponsored. If he *is* grandstanding, he will call for a vote when he knows that he's going to lose. "The way we do it if we want some good publicity," a leading Democratic senator said a couple of years ago, "is to hold hearings on a controversial bill, get all the headlines we can, take a beating on a roll-call vote, and then tell our constituents that we fought the good fight." Although Representative Forand was not considered a highly effective member of the House, no one ever considered him a grandstander, either. "Forand had the one virtue you can't do without in a fight like this—he would never let you down," Cruikshank remarked recently. "Some others might make deals behind your back, but not Forand." Well aware that the conservative coalition that dominated the committee would easily prevail, Forand avoided a roll-call vote on his bill so that he, and all those on his side, could go on building a record.

The immediate effect of the 1958 hearings was that the A.M.A. raised its lobbying budget to a quarter of a million dollars—a fivefold increase. And the Association's staff in Chicago soon began to produce and distribute a vast number of press releases, speeches, and pamphlets attacking the Forand bill. One person who was delighted by this onslaught on the bill was its sponsor. "I am indebted to the American Medical Association for publicizing it so well," Forand said. The debt was considerable. Before the A.M.A. went to work, the bill was almost unknown around the country; within a few months it was being widely discussed.

Everything the A.M.A. did seemed to stir up a furor. Shortly before the 1958 congressional elections, the Chicago office sent the following confidential questionnaire to the top officers of all state and county medical societies:

1. Who is the person or persons in each ward or county in the congressional district who is most influential with the Congress? List the names, addresses, and business or profession of each.

2. Who is the physician who knows and can work with each of the above?

3. Who are the four or five men in the Congressman's district who really influence him? List their names, addresses, and business or profession.

4. Who are the principal contributors to his campaign?

5. What contacts does the medical profession have with officers or leaders of such organizations as the Blue Cross-Blue Shield, dentists, hospital boards or directors, chambers of commerce, farm bureau and grange? Who are the doctors who can talk to these leaders?

6. Who is the Congressman's personal physician at home and in Washington?

7. What contacts does the medical profession have or who knows the Congressman's top secretariat on his Washington staff?

8. What are the Congressman's hobbies, his favorite charities, boards or organizations, church?

9. What papers in the district supported him in his last campaign? What is their present attitude toward him?

10. What contact does the medical profession have with any or all of these newspapers, either directly with the editors or through other influential citizens or advertisers?

11. How big a factor is labor in the district?

12. Do any of the labor organizations deviate from the national labor organizations and for what reason?

13. How big a factor are old folks in his district?

14. What contact has organized medicine or individual physicians with the Congressman?

15. What is his general attitude?

The questionnaire wasn't confidential for long, and Dr. Larson was asked to comment on its propriety. "The purpose was to find out the feeling of the congressman and to be able to give to him in the most effective way the position of the American Medical Association through his own physician, through the local organization of physicians," he said. "I see nothing wrong in that." Not everyone saw eye to eye with Dr. Larson on the necessity of the methods that had been chosen. "Any member of Congress who doesn't know where the A.M.A. stands must be in a coma," an Eastern representative said at the time. Others, in Congress and out, also questioned the advisability of using such methods. An editorial in the *Christian Century*, for example, stated, "Whenever the A.M.A. ceases to be a medical academy and becomes part of the power structure, it can no longer call to its defense the deference, the respect, the affection, and the trust which Americans have traditionally and gladly given to their personal physicians." In the end, the questionnaire made members of Congress more wary of the A.M.A. than they already were, and made the public wonder increasingly about the doctors' claims that they were acting solely in the interest of the people.

The questionnaire had no demonstrable effect on the congressional elections that fall, in which the Democrats gained sixteen seats in the Senate and forty-eight in the House. Since this shift clearly improved the prospects of the Forand bill, the A.M.A.'s House of Delegates was called upon to adopt two defensive measures at a meeting in December. The first was an attempt to encourage the growth of private health-insurance plans, which the A.M.A. had sternly opposed in the past unless they were set up and run by doctors; now a report was presented urging the doctors to look on plans run by laymen with a "judicious, tolerant, and progressive attitude." The delegates set this suggestion aside for study, but a resolution that urged all practicing physicians to lower their fees to the elderly was finally approved, after a good deal of grumbling and wrangling. A number of doctors spoke out against the resolution even after it had been passed; one of them, Dr. Harold J.

Peggs, went as far as to write an article on the subject for *Medical Economics* in which he said, "This gesture is not only futile but downright dangerous."

One of the main purposes of the meeting was to rally opposition to the Forand bill within the profession, and another purpose, not on the agenda, was to keep any likely heretics within the fold. Afterward, Forand reported that a doctor had told him that instructions had gone out "from headquarters of the A.M.A. to the secretaries of the several state societies to pass the word around to doctors, in an inferential way, telling them that if they should testify in favor of the Forand bill they might be violating the ethics of the profession and subject themselves to sanctions."

Some months earlier—on August 19th—Senator Kennedy rose on the floor of the Senate to deliver a speech entitled "A Bill of Rights for Our Elder Citizens," which outlined a program for dealing with the most pressing needs of the aged, including employment, housing, recreation, increases in Social Security benefits, and medical care. A few days afterward, Reidy, who hadn't given up hope of getting a subcommittee on the aging started, had a talk with Ralph Dungan, who was then Kennedy's assistant on the staff of the Labor and Public Welfare Committee. (He is now Ambassador to Chile.) As Reidy explained his idea of setting up a new subcommittee, Dungan became more and more enthusiastic, and from then on he was, as one of his associates has put it, "the senior-citizen man in the Kennedy camp."

By this time Sorensen had come around. Myer Feldman, who was an important figure on Kennedy's staff both in the Senate and in the White House, recalled not long ago, "Sorensen and I worked long and hard on this entire problem throughout 1958. Wilbur Cohen frequently flew in from Michigan so that we could discuss things in detail, and he and I spent many hours, many nights, trying to set up a realistic program. Senator Kennedy was interested in the subject because of the growing number of older people in the population. He felt that Eisenhower had ignored many grave social problems, and that this was one of the gravest. Anyway, we discussed it off and on most of that year, mainly in terms of its social and political impact. We knew it was a big issue and getting bigger every month, and we felt that it could have a very great effect on the outcome of the Presidential election in 1960."

In the fall of 1958, Kennedy was devoting nearly all his attention to getting reëlected to the Senate. A few weeks after the election, he agreed, in the course of a long-distance telephone conversation from Massachusetts, to let Dungan send a letter to Senator Hill in his name requesting that a subcommittee on the aging be set up by the Labor and Public Welfare Committee and that he be made its chairman. As it happened, Hill had received a similar request a few days earlier from Senator Pat McNamara, of Michigan, through *his* assistant on the Labor and Public Welfare Committee, John Sweeney, and since Sweeney had the authority to sign his boss's name and Dungan didn't, McNamara, although lower in seniority, got the chairman's approval. Hill submitted a resolution to the Senate when it reconvened in January, and, on February 6, 1959, he was authorized to set up a Subcommittee on Problems of the Aged and Aging. McNamara was up for reëlection the following year and was badly in need of some publicity. His appointment as head of the new subcommittee provided a handy forum, and he at once collected a small staff and made arrangements for a series of hearings to be held in the coming summer and fall. For the moment, the matter rested there.

Congress had taken no action on the Forand bill in 1958, but it had approved an increase in Social Security benefits, and, to pay for them, had raised the taxable wage base under the program from forty-two hundred dollars to forty-eight hundred. Since an increase in both benefits and taxable wage base had been included in Forand's bill, he was now able to concentrate on health insurance for the aged. As a result, when he introduced his bill in 1959, he was able, by limiting the coverage provided, to reduce the increase in payroll taxes his measure would impose on employees and employers from one-half of one per cent each to one-quarter of one per cent each. In other words, the maximum deduction that could be made from anyone's pay check under the new bill was twelve dollars a year.

One government official who appeared with Secretary Folsom when he testified against the Forand bill during the 1958 hearings was Charles I. Schottland, the Commissioner of Social Security. Now, having resigned at the end of that year, he made it clear that he actually favored the bill. "Here is an opportunity through a relatively small payroll tax—a tax which I believe the American people are willing to pay—to finance the program contemplated," he said not long after leaving office.

Schottland's statement was an example of the political disarray on the issue. "The jerseys were so muddied that you couldn't tell who was on which team," one man who was involved has since remarked. The Republican President was opposed to the bill, and so, at that time, were the Democratic leaders in Congress—Sam Rayburn, the Speaker of the House, and Lyndon B. Johnson, the Majority Leader of the Senate—while the Democratic Advisory Council, whose members included former President Truman and Adlai Stevenson, came out for the bill. Probably nothing illustrated the confusion better than a report on the subject of hospitalization insurance for Social Security beneficiaries that was released by H.E.W. in the spring of 1959. Signed by the new Secretary, Arthur Flemming, the report presented the arguments against the Forand bill and then went on to cite a succession of facts and figures that added up to what looked like a compelling argument for it. (Again to many people's surprise, it was later divulged that Flemming, like Folsom, privately favored the bill, although he was obliged to oppose it publicly.)

Among the new statistics that the H.E.W. report added to the record were the results of a survey that had recently been conducted by the Social Security Administration. This revealed that at that time three-fifths of all the people in the United States over the age of sixty-five had less than a thousand dollars a year in income, while another fifth had between one thousand and two thousand. Of the couples who lived alone in their own homes—the best off among the elderly—nearly half had incomes of less than two thousand dollars a year, and half the elderly who were single and were living alone outside institutions had incomes of less than nine hundred dollars a year. Citing a survey conducted by the Federal Reserve Board not long before, the H.E.W. report pointed out that close to half of all families headed by someone over sixty-five had total assets of less than five hundred dollars. Even so, it went on, "the typical retired couple did not receive income from public assistance, nor did relatives outside the household contribute money to their support."

The self-reliance of the old people who were studied appeared even more remarkable in the light of another fact the report disclosed—that the median income of Social Security beneficiaries who were married came to $2,190 a year per couple (including all outside income), or forty-two dollars a week. Moreover, only three per cent of these married beneficiaries had no medical expenses during the survey year; nine per cent had expenses running to better than eight hundred dollars; and over fifty per cent had expenses ranging from one hundred to eight hundred dollars. "Relatively few—14 per cent of the couples and 9 per cent of the nonmarried beneficiaries—had any of their expenses covered by insurance," the report stated.

The report drew no conclusions from all this, but it left no doubt that about all that an elderly person faced with heavy medical expenses could do after he had exhausted his savings (which, since he was no longer employed, could never be replenished), and perhaps sold his home (only to start paying rent, which would further reduce his assets), was to go on welfare (at a considerable cost to the community, to say nothing of his own pride). There was, of course, one other course open to him: he could put off getting any medical care at all until it was absolutely unavoidable—or too late.

16

THE simplest way to dispute a record that is beginning to look indisputable is to act as if it doesn't exist. Beginning in the late nineteen-fifties, the A.M.A. adopted a new theme—the old people's cause had been taken up by a few cheap politicians and labor leaders whose only motive was to secure their own positions, and there were really no problems of the elderly that could not be handled through existing welfare mechanisms. Around this time, Dr. Edward Annis, a surgeon from Miami, became the A.M.A.'s chief spokesman on public issues. A resourceful debater with a startling ability to produce unanswerable statistics on the spot, Dr. Annis refused to debate other doctors, and insisted on having labor leaders or their friends in Congress as his opponents. This strategy met with some success, for the labor movement had become tainted in many people's minds as a result of revelations of corruption in certain unions. (The Teamsters, led by James Hoffa, had recently been expelled from the A.F.L.-C.I.O.) But the A.M.A.'s primary method of getting around the record and winning support for its views was the old familiar one of lobbying. Over the years the Association had become so thoroughly convinced politicians understood nothing but pressure that it had come to understand nothing else itself.

By and large, the pressure that is exerted most effectively on members of Congress is exerted indirectly. It is thought to be rare for anyone to bribe a member outright. For favors done at the time of a crucial vote, a grateful lobbyist may arrange for a member to lecture before his clients for an inflated fee, but even cases of this sort are believed to be uncommon. An experienced lobbyist won't make any attempt to approach a member who disagrees with him. Any direct pressure on a man who has openly made his stand known is likely to bring what every lobbyist fears most—denunciation on the floor of the Senate or the House and a demand for an official investigation; that alone is enough to put the most influential lobbyist out of business overnight. For the most part, then, lobbyists concentrate on members who are already sympathetic to their views or who are undecided. In these cases, the approach varies. Probably the most common method is to contribute to a man's campaign, or perhaps to lend him the assistance of a couple of public-relations men for a month or two before election time. Off and on in the course of a year, lobbyists write speeches or do research in their field for friendly members. Or they keep their eyes open and warn a legislator about new problems that have come up back home or elsewhere in the government. The most direct pressure they are likely to use, and then only on an important issue, is to persuade a number of the legislator's constituents to flood him with letters, telegrams, and telephone calls. Even then, the lobbyists will do their best to make it appear that the campaign began spontaneously or that someone else was responsible for it.

In the end, a lobbyist's most effective technique is the simplest and most obvious—making a friend of a legislator. "Psychological pressures are far sounder than financial or political pressures," one highly successful lobbyist said recently in the course of describing this technique. "I spend by far the largest part of my time on personal attention. Say, for example, that I'm talking to a senator who is a member of a key committee and I notice that he's coming down with a cold. Well, after I leave I stop off at the nearest drugstore and send a messenger with a bottle of cold tablets to him. Who could accuse me of trying to buy anyone with a dollar's worth of cold tablets? But it's remembered. It's thoughtful. Or say one of his staffers is leaving to take another job back home. I hear about it, and the next time I see the senator I mention what a good egg this fellow is and that I'd like to give him a nice sendoff. How about if I bring a pile of steaks and a case of Scotch to the senator's house and we all have a cookout? After all, the man is leaving, so how could it be considered pressure? But it's another thoughtful act.

"Take an example that happened some time back. I had been building up a relationship with a congressman who's very important to my people, and one day when I was in his office chatting about this and that, he reminded his secretary to clip the foreign stamps off his mail. 'My boy is crazy about stamps,' he told me. A couple of weeks later, I sent the kid some special issues I happened to run across. They only cost five dollars, but that gift was a lot more useful than handing the father a thousand dollars. First of all, if I tried that, he'd probably throw me out. And even if he didn't, he'd be bound to feel guilty and avoid me. But with five dollars' worth of stamps he's grateful and is happy to see me. Besides, later on I can ask 'How is your boy doing with his stamp collection?' as a reminder. I couldn't very well ask 'How are you doing with that thousand bucks?' Slowly, slowly, we become friends, and before long I can come and go at will. If I'm careful, he'll never even realize what's happened. One time, I was standing out in the corridor with a senator I'd become friendly with when a lobbyist for another outfit went by. The senator didn't like him, and when the man was out of earshot he turned to me and said, 'Another lousy lobbyist!' He'd forgotten that I was one, too."

According to several members of Congress who have been on the receiving end, opponents of Medicare have employed all the usual tactics at one time or another. A couple of years ago, one member of the House was overheard saying that a representative of his state's medical society had approached his assistant and offered to make a campaign contribution of ten thousand dollars if the congressman would come out publicly against government health insurance. "That's a good bit of money, especially when I'm not even on Ways and Means," he said. "And a colleague of mine who isn't on the committee, either, but has a few years' seniority on me in the House told me he was offered twenty thousand."

Since the end of the Second World War, organized medicine has been increasingly active at election time—at a cost of many millions of dollars and with very modest results. Of course, the A.M.A. also relies on more subtle methods of persuasion. In an article that appeared in *Medical World News* a couple of years ago, James Foristel, one of the A.M.A.'s Washington lobbyists, was quoted as saying, "We make friends doing little favors. I may help a congressman write a speech. Another may want to know how to get his son into medical school. I tell him how. Still another needs advice on getting his sick wife into a hospital, and I help." Foristel's efforts have not gone unrewarded. "A good example of the kind of attention that pays off," the article went on, "is the experience of Rep. Thomas B. Curtis (R-Mo), one of the A.M.A.'s most powerful allies on the Ways and Means Committee. When he first came to Washington in 1951, his long-time friend, Foristel, temporarily dropped his A.M.A. duties to help him set up his office and get off to a good start. Rep. Curtis has been grateful ever since." But for its most effective lobbying, the A.M.A. has relied on its two hundred thousand members to put its message across—at civic-club lunches, on the golf course, at dinner parties, and, most of all, in their offices and at their patients' bedsides.

17

By THE summer of 1959, the A.M.A. had finally come to see that the Forand bill constituted a real threat. When it was announced, late in June, that the Ways and Means Committee would hold another round of hearings on the measure in July, the Chicago office at once sent each of the Association's members a letter headed "Legislative Alert," which was signed by Dr. Louis M. Orr, the current president. "As you know," Dr. Orr wrote, "this legislation would establish a dangerous and gravely harmful precedent that would undermine the patient-physician relationship and would open the doors to the eventual socialization of medicine." It was urgent, he continued, that each doctor write, wire, or telephone his congressman and Chairman Mills, and get his friends to do the same. Later on, he informed the doctors, they would be given "detailed reasons why [the bill] would be harmful to the nation and to the practice of good medicine."

The A.M.A. also alerted each state medical society and asked for local support. A typical response was an "Emergency Legislative Bulletin" that the California Medical Association sent to its members. Describing the Forand bill as "another socialized medicine scheme," the bulletin went on to say that it was to be "financed by a large increase in Social Security taxes." Since physicians, at their own insistence, were not included in the Social Security program, it was clearly not direct self-interest that prompted the California Medical Association's concern about the "large increase"—of twelve dollars a year at most for salaried workers—in other people's taxes. But a surprisingly frank expression of self-interest was to be found in the bulletin's assertion—an incorrect one—that the

Forand bill would allow the government to "establish the schedule of fees under which doctors will be required to practice."

Secretary Flemming was the first witness at the 1959 hearings. Looking rather uncomfortable, he acknowledged that a problem existed but said that the administration did not feel the Forand bill was an appropriate remedy. Taking the same position that Folsom had taken the year before, he declared that voluntary health insurance should be given a chance. Schottland, the former Commissioner of Social Security, hotly disputed this view. "There is no question in my mind that voluntary insurance can make an even bigger contribution . . . and that it will continue to do so," he testified. "There is also no question in my mind that it cannot be the answer to the total problem of medical care for the aged." Cruikshank was on hand to support this point with some additional facts for the record. He said that the introduction of the Forand bill had frightened the insurance industry to such an extent that some companies had come out with health-insurance policies for the elderly, and he cited as an example a plan offered by Continental Casualty, which, he said, had "flooded the airwaves and newspapers with advertising of a sixty-five-plus policy." Its benefits, he went on, included a maximum allowance for hospital room-and-board charges of ten dollars a day (the going rate was about twenty dollars), a maximum of thirty-one days of hospitalization in any one year, a maximum payment of a hundred dollars for hospital "extras" (which could often equal room-and-board costs), and no provision for nursing-home care. "The vast bulk of health expenditure is not covered at all by this insurance," Cruikshank said.

Once again, Dr. Larson appeared for the A.M.A. After stating that "since 1900 better medical care has increased the life expectancy of the average American by 20.5 years," he went on to say that American doctors had created the problem and American doctors would solve it. Other witnesses pointed out that a number of factors had been responsible for the increased life expectancy, including shorter working hours, earlier retirement, improved sanitation, better food, and the kind of prosperity that made it possible for more people to afford a doctor, not to mention the effectiveness of new drugs and medical techniques that had been developed abroad or by doctors in this country working with public funds.

Another physician to testify against the bill was Dr. Milford O. Rouse, of Dallas, who was at that time the vice-speaker of the A.M.A.'s House of Delegates. (He was soon to become a director of "Life-Line," an extreme right-wing outfit run by H. L. Hunt, the Texas billionaire. At the end of June, 1966, the A.M.A.'s House of Delegates elected Dr. Rouse president of the Association by acclamation.) Dr. Rouse, appearing on behalf of the Texas Medical Association and—so he claimed— "the overwhelming majority of fellow Texans," talked at some length about a study of voluntary health insurance that his state's medical society had made the year before. "They reported for one thing that there were no bona-fide instances of anyone suffering from lack of proper medical care in our good state," he testified. What this statement actually meant was that no one had had to go without a doctor provided he was willing to become a charity case.

Other witnesses testified that even charity care was hard to get in some parts of the country. Walter Reuther, president of the United Auto Workers, said that in many areas welfare applicants had to be able to prove they had been residents for as long as five years. Once that was established, they had to prove they were paupers. If they weren't and still wanted help, the welfare authorities effectively pauperized them by refusing to give any help until they—and, in some jurisdictions, their relatives—had disposed of all their assets. When all those requirements had been met, Reuther went on, medical care was often given "grudgingly and under conditions which make it extremely difficult for a self-respecting person, with a lifetime record of independence, to accept help." Those who went ahead anyway, he said, were likely to find that the care they finally got was second-rate, if not worse. "While some advances have been made in the provision of charity medicine in a way that does not offend the patient," he testified, "the unrelenting struggles of harassed personnel with heavy case loads, insufficient staffs, and inadequate budgets, too often lead to an inescapable erosion of medical standards and a common disregard of the sensibilities of the sick."

A point that didn't come up in the hearings but was later noted by some of those who took part in them was that the A.M.A.'s position on charity medicine seemed to contradict at least two of its other positions—on the importance of what it likes to call "the sacred doctor-patient relationship" and on the importance of the patient's right to choose his own doctor. The A.M.A. could hardly have been unaware that in most charity wards patients were treated by any doctor who happened to be on duty (very often an interne) or that in many institutions there was no guarantee that they would see the same doctor twice—two circumstances that made it difficult for a patient to establish a relationship with a doctor and impossible for him to choose the one he preferred. According to Miss Lisbeth Bamberger, who was Cruikshank's chief assistant in the unions' fight for Medicare, the only explanation for this contradiction was that the A.M.A. made basic class distinctions. "It has one set of standards for those who can pay their bills, and another set for those who can't," she said recently.

In any event, Dr. Rouse's suggestion that proper medical care was universally available was also questioned by some of his colleagues—most explicitly by Dr. Frank F. Furstenberg, medical director of the outpatient department of Sinai Hospital, in Baltimore, where he was in charge of charity patients. Dr. Furstenberg testified:

There is a lot of poppycock about everyone getting medical care who needs it. It depends on the rate at which you get the medical care. If someone comes to an outpatient department or to a hospital emergency room and is in cardiac failure and needs to be hospitalized right away, there are no questions asked. But suppose the person comes in with hypertension and incipient failure, and it looks as though he needs medical care and he is a transient or he is indigent. There are many hospitals that will not take care of such patients until they establish eligibility, go through a means test so that the hospital can collect.

The second round of hearings, like the first, produced no legislation but made weighty additions to the record. They also made more and more people, in government and out, aware of the magnitude and significance of the problem of adequate medical care for the aged. Even so, one A.M.A. official, running true to form, remarked shortly after the hearings ended that most of the problem would be solved if only people didn't retire so early.

18

"A REVOLUTION of rising expectations is in progress in the field of health and medical care," the Joint Economic Committee of Congress reported in the fall of 1959. "Widespread concern about the chronic and degenerative health problems of the aging reflects an awareness of the human and social costs imposed by increases in the older age groups of the American population." Perhaps the most striking example of that concern was the reaction to Senator McNamara's hearings, which were held first in Washington and then in a number of other cities across the country that summer and fall. Reporters in Washington give only cursory attention to most congressional hearings, which tend to be as dull as they are numerous. As a result, the Subcommittee on Problems of the Aged and Aging didn't get much coverage when it held hearings in the capital to take testimony from federal officials, representatives of national organizations, and various health and social-welfare authorities. But when the show went on the road, it got far more attention from less jaded reporters in the cities where public hearings were held—Boston, Pittsburgh, San Francisco, Charleston, Grand Rapids, Miami, and Detroit.

"We knew we had a popular issue, but we didn't realize it would be *that* popular," one of McNamara's staff men recalled later. "The Senator's policy in conducting the hearings was unique, as far as I know. After listening to the experts on both sides, he simply opened up the microphone to anyone in the room who wanted to have his say. Well, the old folks lined up by the dozen everyplace we went. And they didn't talk much about housing or recreational centers or retirement problems or part-time work. They talked about medical care. For the first time, we had these people telling what life was like for them—and letting us know that they were more than a lot of statistics. The upshot was that the hearings got headlines and front-page stories everyplace we went. This gave the movement its first big push forward on the national scene."

In February, 1960, McNamara submitted a report on the hearings to the Senate. Its first recommendation was that the Social Security program be expanded at once "to include health service benefits for all persons eligible" under it. Two Republican members of the subcommittee, Senators Everett McKinley Dirksen and Barry Goldwater, didn't agree with this recommendation, and they submitted a minority report in which they said, among other things, that "the problems of older Americans are basically no different from those of other citizens." Dr. Orr, of the A.M.A., went further. "This is a politically inspired committee," he told the press, and he added that in the course of the hearings "observers heard little support expressed by the older citizens."

The printed transcript of the hearings did not bear out Dr. Orr's statement. Besides those elderly citizens who had stood up to speak for themselves as individuals, quite a few representatives of organized groups had appeared. One of them, the president of the Los Angeles County Senior Citizens Association, which at the time had twenty-three thousand members, stated, "Doctors will tell you that if senior citizens apply, they will give them charity. Now, our senior citizens are independent people. They have a heritage of independence. They do not like to ask for charity. We consider a federal medical-care program the only solution for us on low income." A representative of the Council for the Aging of Springfield, Massachusetts, noted that many old people lived in constant fear that they would get sick and not be able to take care of themselves, and he continued, "A guarantee from Congress that we might retain our independence and not be placed on the charity rolls when our health fails and there is a large drain on our savings would take a lot of worry off the minds of many useful retired citizens."

As an illustration of how disturbing this kind of worry

could be, a doctor from California read the subcommittee part of a note written by a man when he and his wife decided to kill themselves:

> I am sorry that it had to end this way but I see no other way. . . . If you will look over the drug bills you can see that what little money we have could not last long. . . . Last month our drug bill was $83.31. The Thorazine shots for Mary are $1 cash each—sometimes two a day, besides the other medicine. Pray for us that God in his great mercy will forgive us for our act.

A few days after McNamara released his report, some members of the House of Representatives received a list of the doctors in their districts, along with a covering letter from the A.M.A. explaining that the list would enable them to "keep in touch with these physician constituents." The A.M.A.'s friends in Congress were embarrassed, and its enemies were outraged. One of the latter asserted that this was "the most brazen attempt at intimidation I've ever experienced." An even clumsier gesture on the part of the medical profession was made a couple of weeks later when the Chicago Medical Society held a meeting at the Palmer House. Among its "scientific exhibits" was a barker in formal dress and false whiskers standing next to a cash register labelled "Public Till," beside which was prominently displayed a copy of Marx's "Capital." While distributing gold-covered candy coins, the barker chanted, "Step right up and hear about the Forand bill, yes, F-o-r-a-n-d. Don't forget the name, he won't forget you. . . . It's the bill to provide free medical care, free everything, and payola for the U.S. government. . . . Yes, sir, the Forand bill gives you freedom from want, freedom from fear, freedom from freedom." A sign near the exhibit warned doctors that under the bill the government would "take away your older patients and their dependents unless you sign up." When a couple of photographers tried to take pictures of the exhibit, they were forcibly escorted from the hotel by some of the doctors, who explained to reporters outside that the intruders had been sent in by the Communists.

In March, 1960, the Eisenhower administration and the Republican leaders in Congress announced that they were agreed in opposing any health-insurance legislation that was financed through Social Security. "The question of federal aid for medical care of the aged is fast emerging as the most politically significant domestic issue of the election year," Edward T. Chase commented in the *Reporter* not long afterward. "The determination of our next President may be profoundly affected by the debate." One person who was without doubt profoundly affected was Vice-President Nixon. He and Flemming were said to be desperately trying to persuade the President to agree to a bill that would at least take some of the pressure off the Republican Presidential candidate and the Republicans in Congress who were up for election. Nixon's difficulty was increasing every day, for while General Eisenhower kept putting him off, the three leading contenders for the Democratic nomination—Senators Kennedy, Humphrey, and Symington—were publicly calling for passage of the Forand bill. Late in March, the three attended a rally at the State Fair Grounds in Detroit. Kennedy delivered the first speech—a fiery one praising the Forand bill and condemning the Republicans for opposing it. "He was terrific, and he got a terrific response," one of the organizers of the rally recalled later. "I overheard a political columnist tell him afterward that this was going to be the key issue of the campaign. Most of us felt that this was the point where Kennedy became really committed. He went back to Washington and started working on a bill of his own."

Before long, there were almost as many health-insurance bills in the Senate as there were men who wanted to be known as liberals. Nixon returned to the White House to restate his view that neither he nor any other candidate could ignore sixteen million people—around twenty per cent of the electorate. Failing to bring about any change of opinion in the White House, he turned to the Republican members of the Ways and Means Committee and urged them to come up with a modified version of the Forand bill that would be acceptable to him, to the President, and to the A.M.A. "We might have been able to satisfy Nixon and Eisenhower," a Republican member of the committee later remarked, "but, hell, we knew those fellows out at A.M.A. headquarters in Chicago wouldn't accept anything."

By the end of March, mail on the Forand bill was deluging members of Congress, and was running two to one in favor of the measure. As usual in such circumstances, part of the mail was generated by interested organizations—in this case, the A.M.A. and the A.F.L.-C.I.O.—and that part was largely discounted by the recipients, who pay little attention to identically or very similarly worded letters and postcards, however great their number. Much of the mail, though, was clearly spontaneous, such as a note to Senator Jacob Javits, of New York, that read, "I am 80 years old, sixty-four years in industry; sickness has taken my home, insurance policies, and now a pauper's oath, so as to get medical care. Fine thing for a democracy!" The public clamor finally forced the Ways and Means Committee to consent to a vote on the bill on March 31st. The vote was seventeen to eight against it.

Such a lopsided negative vote would ordinarily have meant that the bill was dead—not just for that session but probably for years to come. However, support outside Congress was building up at such a rate that before long the Forand bill's supporters in the House began to talk about bringing it up again. Ten days after the vote, the *Times* noted, "The question of medical insurance for persons over 65 years of age has become one of the hottest political issues in the nation." The next day, a senator said, "Believe me, the heat is on full blast, and we are stewing." By this time, the mail was overflowing the Senate and House post offices, and had reached the astonishing ratio of thirty to one in favor of the bill.

19

As EVERY seasoned politician knows, organized conservatives remember political disappointments far longer than organized liberals do, while the disorganized public forgets them almost at once. During an election year, particularly a Presidential election year, members of Congress hope to find some way to satisfy all three groups—or at least not to offend any of them too seriously. The constituent who has nothing to give or withhold but his vote may be satisfied with some brave words and a promise or two, but the constituent who has campaign funds to offer, influence to wield, and followers to deliver is harder to please. One course of action open to the officeholder when a controversial matter is pending is to assure liberal groups, chiefly labor leaders, that he will go down fighting for their cause, and to assure conservative groups, chiefly businessmen, that he won't act at all unless public demand becomes so pressing that his seat is in jeopardy. Then he will usually appeal to congressional leaders to take him off the hook by postponing action until after the election. And the leaders usually do just that. If they don't and if members are forced to stand up and be counted, most of them will rise on the side of the conservatives, whose bankrolls match their memories.

For these reasons, few men in Congress thought that the Forand bill had any chance of passing in 1960, despite the cataract of mail on the subject. (Among those who were convinced that there would be no action were some of the bill's chief supporters, including Senator Kennedy. "He knew at the time that it couldn't possibly get through," one of his aides said not long ago. "In fact, all the leading men in the Senate knew it.") But on this occasion it soon became clear that the concern of the voters was too deep and abiding to be dealt with in the usual fashion, and in early April both Johnson and Rayburn reversed their former position. Rayburn spoke to Mills, and told him that something had to be done for the elderly voter, and done before election time. Mills was reluctant, but in the end he agreed to let the Ways and Means Committee reconsider Forand's bill. When word of this agreement leaked out, the A.M.A. blamed everything on Reuther, who, it said, had "deliberately misinformed the American people" in an attempt to "stampede Congress."

On May 1st, the *Times* reported that "pressure and heat from the home precincts have brought the issue of health insurance for the aged to the boiling point in Congress." The temperature was still high in the Vice-President's office, too. The White House had finally come around, at least part way, to Nixon's view of the situation and was working on a bill of its own, but it was rumored that Nixon was uneasy about how the public would react to the approach the bill was going to take. It was also rumored that he was prepared to accept a fair degree of me-tooism, but that Eisenhower would not give in. As Chase observed in the *Reporter* at the time, "the issue crystallizes Democratic and Republican ideological differences as do few others."

Early in May, the administration presented its bill, which it called a Medicare Program for the Aged. (This was not the first use of the term "Medicare"; in 1956 Congress had passed an administration measure providing medical care for dependents of servicemen which went by that name.) In many ways, the bill offered far broader medical coverage than Forand's. It provided payment for six months' hospitalization; for the fees of physicians, surgeons, and dentists; for private nursing; for a year's care in nursing homes; and for X-ray and drug therapy. Those eligible were to be single people over the age of sixty-five who had incomes of less than twenty-five hundred dollars a year and couples over sixty-five who had incomes of less than thirty-eight hundred dollars a year; the charge was to be twenty-four dollars a year per person. The plan was to be financed by matching grants from the federal and state governments, totalling a billion and a quarter dollars annually, and the sum was to be used to subsidize insurance policies for the elderly poor that would actually be written by commercial carriers.

At first glance, this bill, based on what looked like an ingenious method of using government funds and yet leaving control of the program to private business, appeared to go a long way toward meeting the needs of the aged. But closer inspection raised some doubts. For one thing, coverage did not begin until the beneficiaries themselves had paid sizable amounts, known as deductibles, out of their own pockets—two hundred and fifty dollars for unmarried participants and four hundred dollars for couples—and, on top of that, the beneficiaries were to be responsible for twenty per cent of all costs above those amounts; in other words, a typical couple with medical expenses of five hundred dollars would be able to collect thirty-two dollars. Moreover, the program would require a much larger staff than the Forand bill, since an entirely new apparatus would have to be set up to deal with the fifty states (each with different legislation regulating use of the new funds) and with over eleven hundred insurance companies (each entitled to a fair share of the business).

The bill attracted few supporters. Governor Rockefeller said that it was fiscally irresponsible and cumbersome to administer; the A.F.L.-C.I.O. said that it was hopeless on every score; the A.M.A. denounced it as government interference; Senator Goldwater called it socialized medicine; and Vice-President Nixon declined to comment on it at all. The President, on the other hand, stood up for the measure—or so it was thought after he commented on it at a press conference: "I am against compulsory medicine and that is exactly what I am against, and I don't care if that does cost the Treasury a little bit more money there. But after all, the price of freedom is not always measured just in dollars." Although no one took the administration's bill seriously, its submission to Congress meant that both parties now accepted the idea that the federal government had an obligation to assist old people who were sick and too poor to pay for medical care. It also meant that some kind of bill was certain to pass before the election.

At that point, all the contestants turned their attention to the Committee on Ways and Means, which had to approve any legislation on the subject, and to Chairman Mills, whose power and influence were to determine the outcome of the contest then and in the years to come. A quiet, impassive man whose ability has always been recognized, even by those who disagree with him, Mills was born and raised in Kensett (a town of less than a thousand people in northeastern Arkansas, not far from Maggot Slough), came East to get a law degree from Harvard, served briefly as a probate judge back in his home state, and was elected to Congress in 1938, at the age of twenty-nine. Twenty years later, he became chairman of the Ways and Means Committee, the youngest man ever to hold the post. In the opinion of many of his colleagues, while Mills is probably the ablest chairman of Ways and Means in history, he is also probably the most cautious member of the House. Some of them put his caution down to a lack of purpose. "He is a man of great intellect and great indecisiveness," one of them has said. "Shakespeare wrote a play about him." Mills's caution is clearly part of his nature rather than a device of political expediency. As the class prophet for his high-school yearbook, he wrote down what he felt would become of his classmates, and then, before submitting the result for publication, took it around to each member of the class to get his approval. According to a reporter who has watched Mills in action in the House for two decades, "Wilbur's idea of a consensus doesn't mean fifty-one-per-cent support, it means eighty or ninety per cent."

In the summer of 1960, there was no doubt that the consensus on the Forand bill was overwhelmingly negative among the members of the Ways and Means Committee— which supporters of the measure began calling the In No Way and By No Means Committee. Undoubtedly, if Mills himself had supported the bill, several other committee members, particularly among the Southern Democrats, would have gone along with him. However, Mills had some fairly compelling reasons for opposing it. For one, his district was staunchly conservative, and in the past couple of years doctors and insurance agents had spent a good deal of time and money on efforts to keep it that way, at least in its attitude toward health insurance. For another, in 1958 Representative Brooks Hays, of Little Rock, to everyone's astonishment, had been beaten after sixteen years in office by T. Dale Alford, a doctor who hadn't even been on the ticket but had won after an eight-day campaign for write-in votes. Although Mills had never been opposed for reëlection, he had always run scared, and after the Hays incident he began to run terrified. Under these circumstances, of course, Mills was anxious not to alienate the officials of the state medical society, who were unusually influential in Arkansas politics. Accordingly, he was said to have promised them that he would oppose the Forand bill, come what may, and they were said to have promised to support him against all comers.

Late that spring, Reuther called on Senator Lyndon Johnson to urge him to endorse the Forand bill publicly, and Johnson said he would be happy to if Reuther would endorse him for the Presidential nomination. Reuther said he was unwilling to commit himself to any candidate at that stage but would keep an open mind, whereupon Johnson, smiling at his visitor's discomfiture, told him that since the bill had to go through the House first, he would do well to talk to Rayburn about it. Reuther did, and Rayburn called Mills, who assured him that the committee was hard at work on the bill and that the old people would surely be taken care of.

A couple of days after that, Reuther was talking with Mills in the corridor outside the Ways and Means Committee hearing room when Rayburn came by.

"Now, you're going to do something about medical care for the old people, aren't you?" Rayburn asked Mills.

"Why, yes, Mr. Sam," Mills said.

"I mean financed through Social Security, like the Forand bill," Rayburn went on.

"That's right, Mr. Sam," Mills said.

A little later, Reuther appeared before the committee to

present a petition, with thousands upon thousands of signa-
tures, urging passage of the Forand bill. Mills told Reuther
that everything was going smoothly. "We left the committee
confident that the Forand bill would be reported out within
the week," one of Reuther's assistants has recalled. "As far as
we were concerned, the battle was won." On June 3rd, however, the committee voted on the bill and, following Mills's
lead, once again rejected it by the same margin of seventeen to
eight. With that formality out of the way, Mills produced a bill
of his own for the committee's consideration. What he proposed was that the medical-vender payments under the Old
Age Assistance program, authorized in 1950 and expanded in
1956, be extended by permitting the federal government to
make unlimited matching grants to the states to provide medical care for the elderly poor—as long as the states came up
with their share. It was not financed through Social Security
like the Forand bill. The measure was quickly approved by the
Ways and Means Committee, and three weeks later it was
passed by the House, by a vote of three hundred and eighty to
twenty-three. One member of the House later described it as a
"hand-washing operation." Another explained that he and a
large number of his colleagues had voted for the Mills bill in
order to get some sort of legislation on the subject, however
inadequate, through the House, in the hope that the Senate
would add something like the Forand bill to it as an amendment, and that a fairly strong bill would emerge from the
joint Senate-House conference charged with reconciling the
two pieces of legislation.

20

ALTHOUGH Democratic strategists knew that there was no hope of getting anything like the Forand bill enacted that session, they also knew that if they tried to get it passed and failed because of Republican opposition, they would have a prime issue for the Presidential campaign—whoever their candidate was. Accordingly, Majority Leader Johnson and Speaker Rayburn announced that Congress would adjourn only temporarily for the Presidential nominating conventions, and would reconvene afterward to consider the most important pending legislation. The Democrats adopted a plank for their platform endorsing the principle embodied in the Forand bill, and the Republicans adopted one for theirs endorsing the principle embodied in the Eisenhower bill.

Unknown to most members of either Party, still another bill was in the works. Shortly after the Ways and Means Committee had acted on the Mills bill, Senator Robert Kerr, Democrat of Oklahoma, who was not only the wealthiest but, in the opinion of many people, the most powerful man in the Senate, determined to settle the issue his own way. In the Senate, the key to action on any health-insurance legislation was held by the Finance Committee, and the key man on that committee was not the chairman, Harry Byrd, of Virginia, who was old and infirm, but Senator Kerr, the ranking Democrat. Senator Paul Douglas once said that "a Social Security expert is a man with Wilbur Cohen's telephone number." Kerr had that number, and he called Cohen at the University of Michigan to get his opinion of the Mills bill. Cohen explained that Mills had consulted him on various occasions about such a bill but that he had not participated in the actual drafting of it, and that, in fact, he had serious reservations about it.

Kerr was up for reëlection that year, and while he wanted to help Kennedy, who had just been nominated in Los Angeles, he also wanted to help himself, and he knew that a bill with his name on it providing for federal payment of part of the medical expenses of the aged would be a great boost to his campaign. But there were difficulties. "If I go all out for Jack, I'll lose a hundred and twenty-five thousand Baptists," he explained. "And if I come out for health insurance under Social Security, I'll lose every doctor in the state." The solution, developed during his conversations with Cohen, was a bill aimed primarily at helping those of the aged who were neither poor enough to qualify for welfare nor wealthy enough to pay their necessary medical expenses—a group that had come to be known as the medically indigent. The help was to take the form of federal grants to match any funds that the states might provide for programs to be administered by the states. Kerr asked Cohen to draft a bill along those lines—keeping an eye on Oklahoma's welfare statutes, so that his state would get at least as fair a share as any other state. Cohen asked whether the A.M.A. would go along with the program, and Kerr said he would take care of that.

In fairly short order, Cohen had worked out a new bill, which incorporated much of the Mills bill—and which provided preferential treatment for Oklahoma *and* Arkansas. After Congress reconvened in August, he flew to Washington to discuss it with two Kennedy aides, Sorensen and Feldman. When Cohen said that neither the Forand bill nor anything like it had any chance of passing that year, Sorensen and Feldman readily agreed with him. Cohen went on to say that if Kennedy and his supporters in the Senate turned things into an either-or situation—either the Forand bill or the Kerr bill—the Senate conservative coalition would in all likelihood choose the milder Kerr bill, and would thereby kill any hope of getting federal health insurance enacted for years to come. On the other hand, if they regarded the Kerr program as a

111

step up the ladder—a way to help the medically indigent, who were one rung away from the bottom—then some form of the Forand approach could be added later to take care of the rest of the elderly. In other words, he said, the two bills should be looked at not as alternatives but, rather, as supplements to each other. Sorensen and Feldman were convinced—and in time, with Reuther's assistance, they convinced Kennedy—that Cohen's view was the realistic one. Cohen had more difficulty persuading some of the liberals in the Senate to go along. Senator Douglas, the leader of this group, disapproved of the strategy, but finally, after several meetings with Cohen, he came around, and the others followed.

Now, with the stage set, Kerr took off for Chicago to meet with the top men in the A.M.A. A highly persuasive man, he used every forensic trick he knew. "He got absolutely nowhere," an associate said later. "The A.M.A. has been shouting for years about how it always supported the Kerr bill. Well, it certainly didn't support the Kerr bill then. Those men wouldn't budge an inch. Kerr warned them that it was either his bill or Forand's sooner or later, and probably sooner. In the end, they did agree not to oppose him outright. But that was as far as they'd go."

On August 13th, the Senate Finance Committee approved Kerr's plan by a vote of twelve to four. The following day, Dr. Larson, who had just been elected president of the A.M.A., announced the results of a survey that Professors James W. Wiggins and Helmut Schoeck, of Emory University, in Atlanta, had conducted in collaboration with sixteen professors from other universities. "An independent national survey just completed by university sociologists emphatically proves that the great majority of Americans over 65 are capably financing their own health care and prefer to do it on their own, without federal-government intervention," Dr. Larson reported. The survey showed that ninety per cent of the elderly who had been questioned could think of no personal medical needs that were not being cared for. Sixty per cent of them said that they were adequately covered by health insurance, and only ten per cent favored government insurance. "This is of the utmost importance to Congress in its current efforts to shape medical-aid legislation for the aged," Dr. Larson said. The survey, whose reliability was not questioned at the time, made headlines all over the country, and copies of it quickly reached the desks of members of Congress. "I was quite impressed by it," one of them said later. "I began to wonder if maybe the record had been wrong before."

On August 17th, Senator Kennedy and Senator Clinton P. Anderson, of New Mexico, introduced a measure that was to replace the Forand bill at the center of the controversy over government health insurance in Congress during the next few years. It was much like the Forand bill but went considerably further; it provided a hundred and twenty days of hospital care, two hundred and forty days of nursing-home care, and three hundred and sixty home visits by visiting nurses each year. At about this time, the A.M.A. placed a full-page advertisement in several big-city papers urging the Senate to pass the Mills bill, and warning that "when government starts telling the doctor how to practice medicine, telling the nurses how to nurse, telling the hospital how to handle its patients—the quality of medical care is sure to decline."

Throughout the following week, the Senate wrangled over the Kennedy-Anderson bill, a McNamara bill, and a Javits bill (this one was a modification of the administration's bill to subsidize private insurance policies), and then, on August 23rd, the Kennedy-Anderson bill, co-sponsored by fifteen senators, came up for a vote. Vice-President Nixon, now the Republican Presidential candidate, was on hand as president of the Senate, but he wasn't presiding. Instead, the *Times* noted, he was "moving about the chamber like a 'party whip,' apparently rounding up votes." Nixon's strategy was clear; he had to defeat the bill sponsored by his rival for the Presidency, for General Eisenhower had promised to veto it if it passed, and such a veto would hand the Democrats the biggest campaign issue they could hope for. Once it was defeated, Nixon could support Kerr's bill, which would not unduly anger the doctors and would cheer up the old people a bit. The strategy was simple, and so were the tactics—keep-

113

ing together the coalition of Northern Republicans and Southern Democrats.

In the end, Nixon and the coalition prevailed, and the Kennedy-Anderson bill was defeated, fifty-one to forty-four. (The bill would almost certainly have received fewer votes if the senators had thought it had any chance; several of the votes in favor of it were said to have been cast by senators who wanted to be in a position to claim loyalty to their liberal backers and at the same time assure their conservative backers that they wouldn't have voted that way if it had counted.) There was no contest over Kerr's bill; it won by a vote of ninety-one to two, the only nays coming from Goldwater and Strom Thurmond, of South Carolina. Two days later, the conference committee agreed to accept the Kerr bill almost intact, and in mid-September the President signed what became known as the Kerr-Mills Act into law.

Although ten million people were theoretically eligible for help under the Kerr-Mills program, the most hopeful estimate of the number that would actually receive help was about two million. "The significant point to know about the medical-aid bill is that there is nothing in it for the average person," Joseph A. Loftus wrote in the *Times*. "This is state charity for the needy, aged 65 and over." Another significant point, not commented on at the time, was that the new law, which was accepted by the Republicans and finally by the A.M.A., did far greater violence to some of the basic principles of both groups than the Kennedy-Anderson bill would have done. In voting for the Kerr-Mills bill, the Republicans, the traditional fiscal conservatives, were voting to spend money out of the Treasury's general fund without providing for any additional revenues to cover it. It was the liberal Democrats, the traditional spenders, who had wanted a pay-as-you-go program that would have left Treasury funds intact. Moreover, the Kerr-Mills bill was a great deal closer to socialized medicine than the Kennedy-Anderson bill. The new law left the structure and machinery of government medical care entirely up to politicians. To be sure, they were state and local politicians, who had always proved to be more respectful to organized medicine than national politicians had, but still they were politicians, and they were in a position to use the new program for their own ends by determining what that care would be like, how much would be paid for it, and who would get it.

Less than a week after President Eisenhower signed the Kerr-Mills Act, newspapers around the country revealed that the survey conducted by Professors Wiggins and Schoeck of Emory University had not been nearly as objective as had been originally reported. Three days before the A.M.A. publicized the results of the survey, it had been presented at the Congress of the International Association of Gerontology in San Francisco, where it was "totally discredited," according to Leonard Breen, of Purdue, a co-director of the section in which it was discussed. Wayne E. Thompson, of Cornell, another participant in the Gerontology Congress, concurred. "It was my opinion, as well as the opinion of other professionals at the meeting, that this work could not withstand professional scrutiny," he said. Subsequently, nine of the sixteen professors who had helped make the survey dissociated themselves from it. One of them, a woman, said she had been instructed to conduct only sixteen per cent of her interviews with people of low income, and in the case of another professor the figure was only nine per cent. Senator Eugene McCarthy, Democrat of Minnesota, a former professor of sociology, denounced the study on the Senate floor, pointing out that the survey had excluded Negroes, everyone on welfare, and all those in hospitals, homes for the aged, nursing homes, and other institutions. The Reverend Joseph P. Fitzpatrick, a Fordham professor who had also participated in the Gerontology Congress, described the Wiggins-Schoeck survey as a study of medical needs that left out "the very people who are most in need of help."

21

AT THE height of the Presidential campaign, the magazines *Medical Times* and *Resident Physician* estimated that doctors favored Nixon over Kennedy by three to one. Yet this support, gratifying as it must have been to the Republican candidate, could scarcely be compared to the so-called rocking-chair vote. Strategists in both camps were busily trying to assess which way that might go, for, as the *Times* noted, "the over-65 vote is considered a political force, extending far beyond such tranquil retirement centers as western Florida and Southern California." Passage of the Kerr-Mills bill had settled some of the dust stirred up that summer, but both candidates began kicking it up again almost at once. Kennedy repeatedly attacked the limitations of the bill and accused Nixon of taking the position that "we cannot afford medical care for the aged." Nixon replied that the bill certainly did not go far enough, and said that in the next session of Congress he would see to it that the Republican administration's plan for "voluntary" coverage was passed.

In scores of speeches across the country and in the television debates Nixon said that the issue was voluntary insurance vs. compulsory insurance—a basic theme of the multi-million-dollar campaign against national health insurance that the A.M.A. had waged between 1949 and 1952. The statement was more rhetorical than substantial. "Voluntary" sounded good, but what it actually amounted to was that the people who most needed health insurance—the poor, the unfortunate, the improvident—would be the last to sign up voluntarily; instead of paying their own way during their working years for medical care after retirement, they would be almost certain to end up as public charges. "Compulsory" sounded bad, but what it actually amounted to was that wage-earners would be compelled to pay a maximum increase in Social Security taxes of a dollar a month. One illustration of the confusing nature of the two terms was that a large number of the "voluntary" plans used in business and industry were really compulsory since employees had to sign up for them when they were hired.

Although the press had apparently grown tired of the subject, and concentrated instead on the candidates' quarrels over the alleged missile gap, President Eisenhower's record, and what to do about Fidel Castro, the candidates themselves spent a great deal of their time talking about the health needs of the elderly. Kennedy, it was later reported, was surprised by the public interest in the subject and talked about it far more often than he had originally intended to. The Democratic Vice-Presidential candidate had the same experience. Not long ago, Mr. Johnson told of listening to taped recordings of four hundred of his 1960 campaign speeches; in each one, he said, he had got the loudest applause when he talked about health insurance for the aged. After the election, there was a good deal of discussion about which group of voters had been most responsible for Kennedy's victory. According to a man who worked at the headquarters of the Democratic National Committee, every bloc that could claim a hundred and twenty thousand votes was trying to take the credit. "From where I sat," he added, "I'd say it was those fellows over in the A.M.A. who put Kennedy in the White House."

The A.M.A. had not done much to help Senator Kerr, although he was reëlected. "After all I did to save the doctors from themselves, I got only twenty-two per cent of their votes in Oklahoma," he told a friend. Concealing his anger from the A.M.A. itself, he assured its top men that he agreed with their theory that stopping the Kennedy-Anderson bill in 1961 might well stop it for good, but he is known to have said privately that some form of national health insurance was inevitable within a few years. A number of the A.M.A.'s friends in Congress who felt the same way advised the Association to make the best deal it could, and settle for a law it could live with. A few weeks after the election, the House of Delegates met for its convention, this time in Washington. In the course of a seminar on implementation of the Kerr-Mills bill, the subject of federal health insurance came up, and this absorbed the attention of most of the delegates. Dr. Ernest B. Howard, who was the assistant executive vice-president of the A.M.A. and was generally considered to be the man in charge of its political operations, told the group that it must hold fast. "The surest way to total defeat is to say, 'We are now going to sit across the negotiating table and see what you will give us,'" he said. "They are going to fight with everything, and I tell you, gentlemen, we have to fight with every resource, right down the line."

22

To MOST members of Congress, politics is the art of the inevitable. Under ordinary circumstances, they would more readily insult the flag than back a lost cause, however worthy. But once it becomes clear that a significant piece of legislation is bound to pass, they are quick to try to modify it to suit their own political needs, or, that failing, to accommodate themselves to it. They have no other choice, for, as Everett McKinley Dirksen, Minority Leader of the Senate, reminded his colleagues the day before he cast his vote for the civil-rights bill of 1964, "no army can withstand the strength of an idea whose time has come." Nor, he might have added, is anything more difficult than the business of bringing an idea to that point—particularly an idea that proposes a radical change in the way the country deals with, or doesn't deal with, its basic social problems. For one thing, Congress has to be inundated with evidence that a great number of people are getting less than their share of the nation's elementary benefits—so much less, in fact, that they are unable to function properly as citizens. Then their needs must be studied and discussed and publicized until lawmakers and voters both have come to feel that the needs are actually basic rights that are being denied. By that time, the deprivation will probably be so widespread and so acute that it can no longer be ignored. When that happens, Congress can be expected to act.

After Senator Kennedy was elected President, an increasing number of influential men in Washington concluded that it wouldn't be long before the time had come for Congress to take action on the idea of government health insurance for the elderly. According to an editorial in *Life* magazine, the dispute over health insurance had been "the hottest political potato" of the election year. Many members of Congress who had found it too hot to handle just before election time and who, after tossing it back and forth during most of that session, had dropped it and passed the Kerr-Mills bill instead, had hoped that by this means they might be able to avoid dealing with the problem indefinitely. They soon discovered that they were no better off than before. Almost no one liked the new law—except its sponsors and the A.M.A., which by this time had come around to supporting it as the best way of fending off anything like the Kennedy-Anderson proposal. An unnamed government official was quoted by the *Wall Street Journal* as having said, "Congress couldn't reconcile its conflicting viewpoints, so it passed the buck to the states." The new program went into effect that October, and it rapidly became apparent that most of the states wouldn't be able to make much use of the federal government's offer to match funds for assistance to the medically indigent, because they were having trouble supporting their own existing welfare programs.

Late that year, President-elect Kennedy made it clear that the buck had come back to Washington when he told reporters that just about the first order of business for his administration would be the enactment of a measure providing health insurance for the aged. Before long, the newspapers began calling the bill Medicare—the name that the Eisenhower administration had given two of its own programs. Whatever the name, it was generally agreed in Washington that the proposal was, in the words of the *Times*, "the greatest social innovation the government has undertaken in a generation."

Eleven days before leaving office, President Eisenhower convened a White House Conference on the Aging, pursuant to a congressional resolution passed a couple of years before. At the time of the resolution, few people had expected that the conference would be held in the middle of a heated debate on the most pressing problem the aging faced, and since the President had firmly opposed any form of compulsory govern-

120

ment health insurance, it was widely assumed that the conferees—around twenty-seven hundred authorities in the field —had been carefully chosen so that a majority would support the administration's views. This assumption was so strong that some experts who had been invited decided to boycott the meeting, and some who did attend announced on arriving in Washington that the deck was stacked. It *was* stacked, but not the way most of the participants thought. Two of the people who *had* thought that the conference might well be held at a crucial time were Secretary of H.E.W. Flemming and Cruikshank, of the A.F.L.-C.I.O. When preparations for the meeting were being made, Flemming called Cruikshank and asked him if he had any ideas about who would make the best chairman. Cruikshank suggested Representative R. W. Kean, of New Jersey, who had been the top Republican on the Ways and Means Committee until he was defeated, that fall, in an attempt to get elected to the Senate. Kean was a liberal, and Cruikshank had twice gone up to New Jersey and persuaded the A.F.L.-C.I.O. people there to support him in his campaigns for reëlection to the House, even though he was a Republican. Kean was not only a liberal Republican, Cruikshank explained to Flemming, but he was extremely knowledgeable about Social Security matters. (Despite his knowledge of the subject, the Republican leadership in the House had passed over him when a subcommittee under the Ways and Means Committee was set up earlier to handle Social Security problems, and had chosen as chairman Representative Carl Curtis, of Nebraska, a lower-ranking member, who was anything but an expert on Social Security; his credentials, however, were strictly conservative.) In the end, Flemming gave Kean the post, and the two men set up the agenda for the conference, which was broken up into a number of groups, or panels, to deal with specific concerns of the aged.

The A.M.A. assumed that Medicare would come before the health panel, and proceeded to stack it with physician-delegates to the conference. However, Flemming had tipped off Cruikshank that Medicare would actually come before the income-maintenance panel, so Cruikshank proceeded to stack *it* with pro-Medicare delegates. When word got out that Medicare was not on the agenda of the health panel, the A.M.A.'s delegates indignantly demanded, through a formal resolution, that it be transferred there. Chairman Kean ruled them out of order. Since most of the panels were stacked with A.M.A. delegates, the doctors then submitted another resolution—to the effect that at the end of the conference, at the plenary session, the delegates be allowed to adopt resolutions in the name of all the conferees. Again Kean ruled them out of order. To the A.M.A.'s dismay, the income-maintenance panel strongly endorsed President-elect Kennedy's view. Shortly afterward, it got even more support when both Marion B. Folsom, President Eisenhower's former Secretary of H.E.W., and Arthur Larson, a former Special Assistant to the President and his favorite political philosopher, got up and did the same thing —which brought headlines around the country. The A.M.A. blamed the outcome on George Meany, president of the A.F.L.-C.I.O., who, it charged, had waged "a reckless campaign of rule or ruin and the public be damned." A more widely accepted interpretation was provided by Chase, in the *Reporter;* he said that the conferees, in repudiating the A.M.A., had given "overwhelming support to the thesis that medical care has become a basic human right."

23

On January 30, 1961, President Kennedy, in his first State of the Union address, told Congress that "measures to provide health care for the aged under Social Security . . . must be undertaken this year." Two weeks later, he sent a special Health Message to the Capitol, in which he appealed for legislative action to deal with "the harsh consequences of illness," and within a few days Senator Anderson introduced the administration's Medicare bill in the Senate, and Representative Cecil King, of California, who had become the ranking Democrat on the Ways and Means Committee after Forand retired at the end of 1960, introduced it in the House. The new Medicare bill provided for ninety days of hospital care (with a maximum deductible—the amount to be paid by the patient —of ninety dollars), outpatient diagnostic services (with a maximum deductible of twenty dollars per service), a hundred and eighty days of nursing-home care, and two hundred and forty home visits by nurses or other health specialists. Its provisions were available to all Social Security beneficiaries sixty-five or older, or about fourteen million people. The annual cost of the bill was estimated at a billion and a half dollars—including federal grants for the construction of medical-school facilities and for loans to medical students, both of which the A.M.A. also opposed. The cost was to be paid for by an increase of one-quarter of one per cent in the Social Security tax on both employees and employers.

The A.M.A. called the Medicare bill "the most deadly challenge" that the medical profession had ever faced, and appealed to its hundred and eighty thousand members for an "all-out" effort to defeat it. A small part of what was expected of them showed up a few days later when a copy of the *AMA News,* a weekly tabloid newspaper containing general medical information and Cadillac advertisements, was sent to each member. A box on the front page called attention to a double-page "advertisement-poster" inside and stated that it was for display in all members' offices. The announcement explained that the poster, which was entitled "Socialized Medicine and *You,*" was "designed as a conversation piece between physician and patient on this important topic." The poster itself (and a leaflet, with the same text, that was later mailed to all members so that it might be handed to patients or sent to them along with bills if the doctor was too busy for conversation) started out by saying, "The time has come for all of us to stand and be counted on the question of Socialized Medicine," and concluded:

> Your freedom is at stake. Freedom is what we all stand to lose. Your freedom to choose the doctor *you believe is best for you.* And your doctor's freedom—his freedom to treat you in an individual way, adapting his knowledge and skills to your particular problems.
> These freedoms are bound to be lost when the Federal Government enters the privacy of the examination room —controlling both standards of practice and the choice of practitioner.
> And lost with these freedoms will be one of the basic principles of our responsibility to you. A principle expressed in the physician's pledge—"*I will hold in confidence all that my patient confides in me.*"

Like all the other health-insurance measures that had been submitted to Congress over the years, the Medicare bill specifically prohibited any restriction of a patient's choice of physician (except that one could not choose a doctor who wasn't properly licensed or who refused to participate in the program, every doctor being free to refuse if he liked), any interference with medical practice, and any control over the doctor (except that no doctor could treat patients in hospitals that were not approved by state health agencies, which have always been run by doctors). Nor did the bill empower the gov-

124

ernment to enter the privacy of the examination room or to pry a patient's confidences out of the doctor's files. Of course, the kinds of treatment and tests given were to be recorded, so that they could be paid for, but that was true of Blue Cross and every other health-insurance program.

In passing, the poster praised the Kerr-Mills plan, to which, as it happened, all the charges it had erroneously levelled at Medicare applied much more accurately. Under the Kerr-Mills plan, patients rarely had freedom of choice, since it was a welfare program, and welfare patients got what they were given—often whichever interne happened to be on duty when they arrived at a hospital. As for privacy, applicants for Kerr-Mills assistance in many states were subject to having their incomes and assets checked, their homes searched for evidence of valuable personal property, and their medical records opened by the lowliest welfare-department clerk. Furthermore, the Kerr-Mills law put control over the medical care it provided firmly in the hands of local and state politicians. "It is incredible that the American Medical Association fails to see that a law based on the insurance principle would be free from the political domination over individual physicians, which is a major feature of the present law," said Dr. David Rutstein, head of the Department of Preventive Medicine at the Harvard Medical School.

Others felt that it wasn't at all incredible, since the A.M.A. was far less interested in what it always talked about than it was in what it never talked about. Probably the best explanation for the Association's fear of a federally administered insurance program was offered by Chase in a speech he delivered before the City Club of Cleveland at about that time. Chase pointed out that Medicare included a fee schedule for hospitals, nursing homes, and nurses. "And it is here that we come close to the heart of organized medicine's rejection of the Social Security approach," he said. "Even so limited an instance of a fee schedule as this, for government-paid medical services to the retired aged—and the administration's bill does not include physicians' services, incidentally—panics the medical leadership. They anticipate a time when doctors'

125

services will be covered and hence a fee schedule will be used."

Convinced that its vast and expensive publicity campaign of the early nineteen-fifties had defeated President Truman's proposal for national health insurance—which no one else, including the President, had believed had any chance of being enacted—the A.M.A. now announced, late in February of 1961, that it was preparing a similar campaign against Medicare. It was an effort that many people in Washington considered as futile as the earlier one had been unneccessary. "Whether this particular bill or one like it gets through this year or not, no organized force is going to prevent any large segment of the public, such as the elderly, from getting adequate medical care and getting it in a dignified, humane, efficient way," Chase said at the time. "Americans are ingenious and insistent in achieving what they consider their basic social rights." A Democratic member of the House who also believed that passage of federal health-insurance legislation was inevitable remarked that the leaders of the A.M.A. probably believed it, too. "Back in 1949, they levied dues on their members for the first time—twenty-five dollars a head per year—to fight Truman," he said. That brought in between three and four million dollars annually. And now the dues are up to thirty-five dollars. I wouldn't be at all surprised if some of those fellows in the A.M.A. hierarchy got to like having all that money around, considering what it must have done to build up their power." (Later, the dues were raised to forty-five and then to seventy dollars a year.)

The A.M.A. hierarchy and representatives from all the state medical societies held a special two-day meeting in Chicago a month after the King-Anderson bill was introduced. Conducted in strict secrecy—a squad of private policemen made sure that all outsiders stayed outside—the meeting was devoted largely to a discussion of the A.M.A.'s plans for its all-out effort. Various materials were passed around, including a thick "Do-It-Yourself Kit," which was later distributed in bulk to the Association's two thousand state and county medical societies. Among the items it contained were "fact sheets"

126

that defended the Kerr-Mills program and attacked Medicare on statistical grounds; speeches for delivery to medical audiences; speeches for delivery to non-medical audiences; press releases announcing that the speeches had been delivered; one-minute radio advertisements; reprints of favorable editorials, articles, and public statements; sample letters-to-the-editor for local papers; advertising mats; leaflets, posters, and booklets; instructions to the women's auxiliary (doctors' wives) on how to conduct a letter-writing campaign that would produce three-quarters of a million letters to Congress by the end of the year; and descriptions of the best ways to line up support among influential organizations and citizens on the local level.

Also on display was a full-page advertisement that the A.M.A. had scheduled for appearance in twenty-nine large-city newspapers the following month. At the top was the statement "Speaking for 180,000 physician-members, the A.M.A. believes you deserve to know exactly where we doctors stand on the question of: Medical Aid for the Aged." Below, the advertisement proceeded to praise the Kerr-Mills program on the ground that its "benefits are unlimited" (which would have been true if all states had made unlimited services available, but not one of them had), that it was "being put into operation in 46 states" (it was actually in operation in nineteen states, and the figure is still under forty-six), and that it "avoids waste of tax dollars" (it was financed out of general tax revenues, while Medicare was self-supporting). As for the administration's plan, the A.M.A. found it unacceptable because it was "compulsory" (its only compulsory feature was a tax increase of less than eighteen dollars a year) and because its benefits were available to everyone under Social Security, "regardless of need" (like Social Security itself). Unaccountably, the advertisement left out some of the A.M.A.'s favorite claims—that, like the British National Health Service, Medicare would be ruinously expensive, widely unpopular, and medically inferior. However, these points were covered in some of the other material distributed at the meeting and were widely used in the campaign that followed.

Later in 1961, a group of A.M.A. officers met at the Drake Hotel in Chicago to hear William Demougeot, a professor in the Speech Department at the North Texas State University, present an evaluation of their publicity. Assuring them that he was opposed to federal health insurance, he said, "I *want* you people to win your fight." However, he warned them, they might lose it if they were not more careful about what they said and where they said it. Charges that Medicare amounted to socialized medicine were "a big help in prejudicing the public," he went on, but they had best be used sparingly and never with "sophisticated people." The denial of free choice was also useful, but, again, only with an audience that didn't know the facts, because, he said, "it simply is not true." The best way of putting opponents at a disadvantage, Professor Demougeot said, was through the assertion that Medicare would be compulsory. "Sociologists and economists can demonstrate that a national compulsory system is justifiable and probably cheaper, but it's a difficult line of reasoning to present," he explained.

When Professor Demougeot got around to the claim about the British system, he said, "You'd better not use it if you have an audience, or an opponent, who knows how foreign systems are run." Pointing out that in England both patients and doctors had complete freedom of choice, he went on to cite a Gallup poll showing that sixty per cent of the doctors and nearly ninety per cent of the patients were quite happy with the system. The A.M.A. had often charged that the National Health Service had reduced England, medically, to the second rank. The statement was not entirely accurate, he said, because while England *was* in the second rank, it hadn't been even as high as that before the program was adopted. He also pointed out that statements about the exorbitant cost of government health insurance as opposed to private health insurance were difficult to justify. In the United States, the administrative costs of private group plans ran as high as twenty-five per cent of premiums, while in England the administrative costs were around twelve per cent, and, he added, "Their percentage is going down while ours is rising." He also advised the doctors to steer clear of statements about how much it cost to run our Social Security system, because its administrative costs were only six per cent. (On this point the Professor was wrong; the costs were two per cent.)

"I wonder if it has ever occurred to the members of this audience that the United States is the only major nation in the world that does *not* have a national compulsory system of state payment for medical care," he continued. "If the system is really as bad as it is usually pictured here, would fifty-nine nations have adopted it? Wouldn't the conservative party in some nation rally all those discontented people to its cause by proposing to abolish that low-quality, high-cost system?" Still another argument that he felt was "not worth using against an intelligent opponent" was that American medicine was the best in the world and had been made that way through free enterprise and private practice. That was no reason for not making it better, he remarked, and went on to point out, as some witnesses had in the Forand-bill hearings, that the country's physical well-being was also due to improved standards of food, shelter, clothing, and sanitation, and to the fact that most people had more money available to pay for a doctor's services than they used to have. Almost every advance in medicine had been made by a doctor working on salary, he continued, and, furthermore, that salary was often paid by the government. Despite all this, American medicine still wasn't the best in the world—at least, not by some standards. Not only did a number of other countries have a higher longevity rate and a lower infant-mortality rate, Professor Demougeot said, but "the nations ahead of us have one thing in common—the national government pays for medical care."

24

LATE in the spring of 1961, the *Medical Tribune* reported that eighty-one per cent of the doctors were against Medicare, and that summer a Gallup poll showed that sixty-seven per cent of the lay voters were for it. "It was clear then what the outcome would be," said Representative John D. Dingell, Jr., Democrat of Michigan, whose father had co-sponsored the old Wagner-Murray-Dingell bill as well as the first bill for health-insurance for the aged. "It was a case of the doctors versus the people. Naturally, the people were going to win." For the moment, though, it appeared that the doctors were winning. Despite the President's call for action on the King-Anderson bill, it was locked fast in the Committee on Ways and Means, and Chairman Mills still seemed determined to prevent it, or anything like it, from reaching the floor of the House.

While the King-Anderson bill's supporters in Congress mustered their forces for an attack on Mills, the A.M.A. went on trying, as it had for twenty-five years, to keep its allies in line and, if possible, to attract new ones to its cause. Back in February, the A.M.A. had unexpectedly been rebuffed by the General Board of the National Council of Churches, which endorsed the Medicare bill. Afterward, it was generally assumed in religious circles that the United Presbyterian Church would second the endorsement when its General Assembly met in June. As June approached, the delegates to the assembly—there were nine hundred of them—became the object of an astonishing amount of attention from local medical societies, chambers of commerce, business and civic groups, prominent members of their churches, and, often, their personal physicians. It was, the *Christian Century* reported later, a "tremendous, amazingly well-organized, and well-financed" campaign. It was also an effective one. As the magazine put it, "a pressure group barked and the church retreated." The retreat consisted of a refusal to take any stand at all beyond referring the question to a committee for further study.

Not long afterward, the Young Women's Christian Association announced that it supported Medicare, whereupon the A.M.A. sent an indignant letter, expressing "shock" at the decision, to the Y.W.C.A.'s board, which, it declared, was unqualified to judge "such a controversial, technical issue." The ladies were made of sterner stuff than the churchmen, and stood fast. The A.M.A. had also been having trouble with another group of women—a hundred and seventy thousand of them, who made up the membership of the American Nurses' Association. Shortly after the A.N.A. endorsed Medicare in 1958, thirty-five of the nurses' state societies reported that doctors had made various efforts to change their minds, including threats of reprisal against office or hospital nurses who retained their membership in the national organization and offers to pay all the expenses of any nurse who wanted to take a trip to Washington (and publicly express her disapproval of the bill while she was there).

The American Hospital Association—which had always gone along with the doctors up to that time—had officially stated, also in 1958, that some kind of federal health insurance might ultimately be necessary. Now it was rumored that a good many of its members had concluded that the ultimate was at hand. The A.M.A. moved in quickly to suppress the revolt. Hospital staff physicians, hospital trustees, and heads of local chambers of commerce that participated in hospital fund-raising drives began dropping in with surprising frequency to chat with hospital administrators. One administrator, a member of an important committee in the A.H.A., heard from twenty graduates of the medical school that was affiliated with his hospital; each of them threatened to stop contributing to the school if he took the wrong stand at the next A.H.A. meeting. "I didn't feel so intimidated when I checked up and found out that none of them had been making contributions anyway," he said later. When the administrators met to consider the issue, the A.M.A. increased its pressure. "The heat was terrific," a delegate has recalled. "If it hadn't been for all that lobbying, I think we would have gone for a flat endorsement of Social Security financing. As it was, we had to fudge the issue." Like the Presbyterians, the hospital administrators ended up by endorsing nothing. But they did issue a statement noting that federal help of some sort had to be given to the elderly poor, and adding, "The tax source of funds is of secondary importance to us." The statement was not at all to the A.M.A.'s liking, but it put on a brave face and said that it was "gratified" by the hospital administrators' stand.

During the same period, the American Public Health Association, representing forty thousand public health specialists, approved a resolution in favor of Social Security financing for health care. Around that time, too, a growing number of doctors began to break away from the A.M.A.—with a maximum of publicity. In the San Francisco area, two young physicians who objected to statements contained in some one-minute radio spots that had been sponsored by the local medical society paid for twenty-eight one-minute announcements of their own to refute their colleagues. Then they founded the Bay Area Committee for Medical Aid to the Aged through Social Security, and soon signed up two hundred doctors and a thousand laymen. The number of doctors who turned out surprised them, until they learned that the recruits had had no idea of what the provisions of Medicare actually were until they heard the radio rebuttals; when they found out what the bill contained, most of them concluded that it was far too modest to meet the pressing public needs.

Ultimately the founding of this committee and a similar but smaller one in Chicago led to the establishment of a national organization—the Physicians Committee for Health Care for the Aged through Social Security. The members of the national organization included Caldwell B. Esselstyn, president of the Group Health Association of America, who served as chairman; David P. Barr, chief physician at New

York Hospital; Walter Bauer, head of medical services at Massachusetts General Hospital; Martin Cherkasky, director of Montefiore Hospital; Leona Baumgartner, New York City Commissioner of Health; Ray E. Trussell, New York City Commissioner of Hospitals; Arthur Kornberg and Dickinson W. Richards, Nobel laureates in medicine; Benjamin Spock, the pediatrician; Helen Taussig, one of the developers of the blue-baby operation; and Michael E. DeBakey, the heart surgeon. Shortly after the committee was set up, it sent an advertisement stating its principles and its purpose to the *Journal* of the A.M.A. The ad was turned down as "misleading."

25

THOSE who hope to control the events of history in Washington must first understand that the process of gaining, and keeping, political power is an extraordinarily complex one. Men who have reached the top in other fields often find themselves completely outclassed when they enter public life, for politics requires a unique intellectual and emotional capacity. The successful politician devotes years—with a prudent investment of his influence here and an occasional well-considered plunge on a vote there—to accumulating a nest egg of power that will then accumulate substantial interest from the seniority system. Because power is so hard to come by, clever politicians seldom risk it in any large measure. A financier can lose a million dollars and make it up within the week, but a politician who suffers a comparable reverse is faced with political bankruptcy. (In the past hundred and twenty-five years, only one defeated nominee for the Presidency came back to win the office, and that was Grover Cleveland, who had already been President.) In short, when a man loses in politics, he loses big. And the same thing may be said of organizations that hope to wield power in Washington.

In the summer of 1961, the A.M.A.—either overconfident of its strength or unaware of the dangers involved—decided to enlarge its all-out effort against Medicare by participating in the next year's congressional campaign. Since it could not, under federal law, engage directly in a political campaign without endangering its tax-exempt status, an independent group was set up with a contribution from the A.M.A. of fifty thousand dollars—for "educational" purposes, which the law permits. This new organization was called the American Medical Political Action Committee—or, as it came to be known, AMPAC. The A.M.A.'s board of trustees chose the directors of AMPAC, and chose all Republicans until someone pointed out that this meant writing off the entire South. With that, AMPAC became bipartisan, although the bipartisanship had its limits, as one of the directors indicated by publicly stating, "We are out to elect conservatives." As a part of its fund-raising activities, AMPAC published a newsletter, called *Political Stethoscope*, that appealed to all doctors to make contributions, or at least become members. "If we want to keep politics out of medicine, we must get into politics," wrote AMPAC's chairman, Dr. Gunnar Gundersen, who was a former president of the A.M.A. Dr. Gundersen went on to tell his colleagues that "the dollars you use for political purposes may well mean more to your children and your family's future than any other investment you will ever make."

The political campaigns that organized medicine had participated in between 1949 and 1962 not only had failed much more often than they had succeeded but had drawn a good deal of criticism from the public at large because of the outlay of money involved, which was enormous, and the tactics employed, which were often questionable. To avoid this kind of criticism, AMPAC conducted its affairs pretty much in secret, although from time to time its members were unable to refrain from boasting about their accomplishments, and even their expenditures. "AMPAC officials are closemouthed about the size of their membership and campaign kitty," the *Wall Street Journal* reported several months after the organization went into action. Before long it became apparent that AMPAC was thriving. Within a year, forty-six state medical societies had set up their own local political committees, which were autonomous but contributed part of the donations and membership dues they collected to the national headquarters. In return, the national headquarters supplied them with campaign literature, advice on precinct organization, instructions about voter-registration drives, and suggestions for getting out the vote on Election Day. In addition, a special AMPAC squad toured the country and held seminars to teach local groups of

135

doctors some of the more refined techniques of political campaigning and advise them on handling local problems.

Half the doctors in Iowa enrolled in the Iowa Physicians Political League, which turned over forty per cent of its dues to AMPAC. The Texas Political Action Committee asked all doctors in the state who had been in practice for five years or more to take out sustaining memberships in AMPAC, and it was said that two-thirds of them complied; a single fund-raising dinner in Texas produced eighteen thousand dollars for AMPAC. The Indiana Health Organization for Political Education, or I-HOPE, enrolled a thousand doctors, who contributed fifty thousand dollars, and a hundred and twenty of its members spent additional sums in attempts to become delegates to the state conventions of both political parties.

In July of 1961, the same month that AMPAC was set up to oppose Medicare, another group was set up to support it. Called the National Council of Senior Citizens, it was built around the remnants of the Senior Citizens for Kennedy, which had been organized for the 1960 campaign, with Forand as its chairman. Because he himself was elderly and in poor health, he could only be as active in the Medicare fight as his physical condition permitted. At the White House Conference on the Aging, Forand had got into a discussion with several union leaders who were considering whether it was desirable to organize older people to work for Medicare. Some of the men he talked with, such as Cruikshank, opposed the idea, on the ground that it might well lead to a kind of Townsend movement. "The Townsend people, back in the thirties, were wildly irresponsible," Cruikshank explained not long ago. "If they'd had their way, the United States would have been bankrupt inside a year. I was afraid we might create a sort of gerontocracy that would plague the government for one handout after another. We just couldn't get tied up with anything like that."

Two men who ran programs for retired workers in A.F.L.-C.I.O. affiliates—Charles Odell, of the United Auto Workers, and James Cuff O'Brien, of the United Steelworkers—decided in the summer of 1961 to go ahead with the project on a part-time basis, despite the opposition of Cruikshank and other labor leaders. They persuaded their unions to put up small amounts of money, prevailed on Forand to lend his name as chairman, and, as the National Council of Senior Citizens, set up a modest office in Washington with a staff of three. Forand had never got around to answering some six thousand letters from old people who had written to thank him for his efforts on their behalf; now he sent each of them a form letter asking them to join the council and to bring their friends and neighbors along. The idea caught on among the elderly as quickly as AMPAC had among doctors, and within a few months the council had half a million members, a monthly newsletter, and a sizable debt.

The Democratic National Committee completed its analysis of the 1960 election toward the end of 1961, and found that elderly voters had contributed significantly, and in some key districts decisively, to Kennedy's victory. Convinced by this that the new council could be helpful in the forthcoming campaign for Medicare, the National Committee started giving it small donations at intervals to keep it going. About the same time, Cruikshank's associates persuaded him that the best way to keep the council on the right track, now that it was running, was to contribute to its upkeep. (Over the next five years, the council's total budget was about half a million dollars, supplied in more or less equal parts by the Democratic National Committee, the A.F.L.-C.I.O., and individual members, who, if they could afford it, paid dues of a dollar a year.) With funds available, the council was able to hire someone to run it full time. The man who got the job was William R. Hutton, a naturalized immigrant from Great Britain who had been a foreign correspondent for the London *Daily Mail*, a heavily decorated colonel in the British Commando forces, director of the British Information Services for Central Europe, and a New York public-relations man. "When I came down here, it was a bucket-shop operation," Hutton has recalled. "The office was a dilapidated flat, the one secretary worked at the kitchen table and kept the press releases in the bathtub, and there was precious little in the way of funds. The A.M.A.

had all the money, and we had all the old people. My job was to switch them from the bingo circuit to social action."

President Kennedy was also impressed by the analysis of the election returns, and after discussing the matter with members of his staff he decided to make a push for passage of the Medicare bill in 1962. "With a pivotal congressional election coming up this fall," the *Times* noted a little later, "it was patent the Democrats hoped to claim a major achievement if the bill passed, or a campaign issue with real bite if it failed." The stakes were very high. Kenneth O'Donnell, a special assistant to the President, and Richard Maguire, a top man on the Democratic National Committee, were convinced—and they convinced President Kennedy—that the Medicare issue was the only thing big enough to cut down the losses that the party in power normally suffers in off-year congressional elections. The Kennedy administration was having great difficulty in getting most of its program passed, and it was clear that if the Party lost heavily that fall, there would be almost no chance of getting anything at all through Congress.

The news that the President was determined to press hard for enactment of Medicare produced a good deal of excitement in medical circles. Early in January, 1962, just after Congress convened, the Blue Cross Association announced that it had made "a historic decision . . . to finance a program of comprehensive health-care benefits for the aged," that the program was all arranged, and that nothing remained to be done except to translate it into "technical language." Since Blue Cross had always been sensitive to the views of the American Hospital Association, and the American Hospital Association had always been sensitive to the views of doctors, whom it had to get along with on a day-to-day basis, it was generally taken for granted in Washington that the A.M.A. had suggested the idea. Whatever the source of the program may have been, Blue Cross seemed to encounter extraordinary difficulty in translating it into technical language, for the benefits never appeared. The headlines that the announcement created across the country may have momentarily tempered the public demand for enactment of Medicare, but they did not allay the A.M.A.'s strong fear that the bill would be passed before AMPAC could show its strength at election time.

To forestall action in Congress, the A.M.A. and AMPAC stepped up their campaigns. The women's auxiliary was the first to attack. In a program called Operation Coffee Cup, thousands of doctors' wives held afternoon parties for friends and neighbors, at which they ate cookies, drank coffee, and listened to a recording of a talk by Ronald Reagan. "One of the traditional methods of imposing statism or Socialism on a people has been by way of medicine," Reagan assured his listeners, and he urged the ladies to write letters, and get their friends to write letters, to members of Congress. "If you don't do this," he said, "one of these days you and I are going to spend our sunset years telling our children and our children's children what it once was like in America when men were free." Sample letters were printed on the jacket of the record, and after it was played, the hostess passed out pens, writing paper, preaddressed envelopes, and stamps. Around the same time, the A.M.A. speakers' bureau sent seventy of its members around the country to talk to anyone who would listen, and thousands of clubs, fraternal societies, veterans groups, and business and civic organizations did.

All over the country, individual doctors joined the assault. In Indiana, eleven members of the Clinton County Medical Society—its total membership—prevailed on five hundred fellow-citizens to write to their congressman. And downstate, in Corydon, six doctors spent four days canvassing each of the town's thousand homes. In West Virginia, a group of doctors placed a full-page advertisement in the Wheeling *News-Register* asking "Are Doctors Crying Wolf?" Professor Demougeot's advice had apparently not reached West Virginia, for their answer was "The Socialist Party Doesn't Think So! Authorities in England Don't Think So!" While the King-Anderson bill amounted to socialized medicine, the advertisement charged, "by contrast, the existing Kerr-Mills program can provide free-choice, comprehensive care to those in need." One state that had tried to see that its program did provide that sort of care was West Virginia, and it had nearly gone bankrupt doing it. According to an account given by Murray Kempton, in the New York *Post*, "West Virginia seems to have made the mistake of trusting its state medical society." Under its Kerr-Mills program, the state provided for an extra ten-dollar fee for specialists; overnight it seemed that most of the doctors in West Virginia had become specialists. The program allowed thirty days of hospital care at a cost of thirty-five dollars a day; a surprising number of patients had illnesses that lasted exactly thirty days. The program also paid for all drug prescriptions; one doctor who dispensed his own medicine collected thirteen hundred dollars in one month for drugs. In the end, West Virginia had to cut its program in half and reduce doctors' fees drastically. Of the eighteen hundred doctors in the state, Kempton reported, only a hundred and thirty-two stayed in the program after that.

26

EARLY in 1962, the National Council of Senior Citizens announced that it would hold a rally of elderly people in Madison Square Garden in May, and in March the White House revealed that the President would speak at it. The administration's timing gave the A.M.A. two months to devise ways of countering the effect of the rally. It appeared that something impressive would be required, for early in May word leaked out that at a White House breakfast for Democratic congressional leaders the guests had told President Kennedy they had found a groundswell of public support for Medicare during the Easter recess. "Prospects for favorable congressional action . . . have shifted from bad to good in the last few weeks," the New York *Times* reported. Alarmed by this news, the A.M.A. mounted a vast advertising drive during the week before and the week after the President spoke. In that period, thousands of daily and weekly newspapers around the country carried anti-Medicare advertisements, which had been prepared in mat form by the A.M.A. and placed by local medical societies.

A typical advertisement declared, "Surveys show that relatively few of the aged are in poor health . . . [and] that those over 65 are in better financial circumstances than other age groups." These were the Wiggins-Schoeck surveys, which had been prepared for the A.M.A. before the 1960 election and discredited at the time by professional sociologists, including some who had actually worked on the surveys. Another advertisement charged, "The plan would overcrowd hospitals through overuse . . . with throngs of people with minor complaints, imaginary ailments or a desire for a checkup and a day off." Later, Representative King remarked of this argument, "If the A.M.A. expects an increase in unnecessary hospitalization, it must subscribe to the view that physicians are either collaborating with their patients in unethical practices or are unable to make proper medical judgments."

On the afternoon of May 20th, a Sunday, President Kennedy stood before a capacity audience of twenty thousand old people in Madison Square Garden, smilingly accepted their long and enthusiastic welcome, and then put aside his prepared text to deliver one of the worst speeches of his career. At the time his limousine arrived at the Garden, he had been seen scribbling with his silver pencil on a yellow legal pad—making a last-minute attempt to write his own speech, it was learned, because he was dissatisfied with the one that had been prepared for him. But time was running out, since arrangements had been made for national television coverage to begin at precisely four o'clock, so he decided to speak extemporaneously. "It was a fighting stump speech, loudly delivered and applauded," Theodore Sorensen observed later. "But the President had forgotten the lesson of the campaign that arousing a partisan crowd in a vast arena and convincing the skeptical TV viewer at home require wholly different kinds of presentation. He already had support from the senior citizens; he needed more support from the home viewers, and that speech did not induce it."

Down in Washington, the A.F.L.-C.I.O. people who had been working for Medicare watched the televised speech with mounting dismay, which finally turned into despair. "We didn't know it was merely a miscalculation on Kennedy's part," one of them said later. "We thought the President didn't care, that he wasn't really behind the bill at all. Otherwise, how could he have given such a terrible speech? All of us had looked forward to the occasion as the first big opportunity to unite the elderly, arouse the general public, and create an overwhelming consensus. But instead of steam for the Medicare pistons we got a pail of cold water."

The A.M.A. demanded equal time on television to present

its case, but the networks turned it down, so it bought half an hour of prime television time on May 21st and rented Madison Square Garden, too, the total cost coming to an estimated hundred thousand dollars. (The National Council of Senior Citizens and its affiliate the New York Golden Ring Council paid the rent for the Garden by charging a dollar a seat). The A.M.A.'s TV presentation, which was produced by the Troy-Beaumont Company, of New York, opened with a shot of the crowd leaving the Garden the day before, and then switched to the littered arena inside as an offstage announcer said, "The empty seats calmly await the next event. . . . But right now these seats are yours. There will be no pageant. But there will be an appeal to you from physicians of America." The appeal was made by Dr. Edward Annis, the surgeon from Miami who had by this time become the head of the A.M.A. speakers' bureau. He had also become known as the most indefatigable opponent of government health insurance since Dr. Morris Fishbein.

Dr. Annis began by saying that he had been asked whether he would feel foolish addressing an empty auditorium, and that he had replied, "I'm not a cheerleader. I'm a physician." Of the President's address, he said, "These people know how to rally votes, rally support, rally crowds and mass meetings. That's quite a bit of machinery to put behind something, isn't it? Who can match it? Certainly not your doctors. . . . Men and women of America, I appeal to your sense of fairness! Nobody—certainly not your doctors—nobody can compete in this unfamiliar art of public persuasion against such massive publicity, such enormous professional machinery, such unexplained money, and such skillful manipulation!"

Going on to warn his listeners that "doctors fear that the American public is in danger of being blitzed, brainwashed, and bandwagoned," he then brought up the Kerr-Mills program, which, he declared, had "already been accepted by thirty-eight states," and said, "Why aren't you hearing more about it? It works!" (One place where it didn't work was Dr. Annis's home state; Florida was not participating in the program. The following month, a Senate report on the Kerr-Mills

143

program showed that it was working not in thirty-eight states —already a mysterious decline from the A.M.A.'s claim of forty-six states the year before—but in twenty-four. Of these, New York, Massachusetts, Michigan, and California were getting ninety per cent of all the federal funds being distributed —chiefly because they were the only states able and willing to match government grants in any significant amounts. Where the Kerr-Mills program was operating, the report continued, it was usually operating in a very limited way. In March, a total of eighty-eight thousand people, or about one-half of one per cent of the country's aged population, had received some form of assistance, and more often than not the assistance hadn't amounted to much. For instance, Kentucky provided six days of hospital care, but only for "acute, emergency, and life-endangering conditions;" Oregon provided fourteen days, but the recipient paid seven dollars and a half a day for the first ten days; and Idaho provided fourteen days, but only for critical cases. All twenty-four states required means tests, under which applicants qualified only if their annual incomes were less than a certain amount, ranging from a low of a thousand dollars, in South Carolina, to a high of eighteen hundred dollars, in New York. In half the states, means tests were also given to the applicants' relatives.)

Once Dr. Annis had finished praising the Kerr-Mills program, he turned to the King-Anderson bill. Holding up a copy of it, he read the official title—"The Health Insurance Benefits Act"—and asked, "Is it genuine insurance?" Answering himself, he said, "No, it is not. The Supreme Court has held more than once that the Social Security system is not an insurance system." (The A.M.A. was extremely fond of this allegation, which may have planted in some people's minds a suggestion that the government could take payments from those covered under Medicare with no legal obligation to pay out any benefits. Actually, the only statement that the Supreme Court had ever made on this subject appeared in a decision handed down in 1960, which said, "The Social Security system may be accurately described as a form of social insurance, enacted pursuant to Congress's power to 'spend money in aid of the general welfare.' ")

As for the bill itself, Dr. Annis was particularly concerned over a provision in it requiring any hospital that participated to set up a "utilization committee" to review the records of all Medicare patients who had been hospitalized for more than thirty days. "If your illness required hospitalization for more than thirty days, it'd have to be passed on by a special committee who'd have to consider a lot of other people, too, don't ya know," Dr. Annis's script read. "After all, the government has to treat everyone fair and equal, don't ya know. They know all about how to make things exactly alike—like human illnesses. Like a broken toe and cancer. A bed is a bed. Thirty days is thirty days. Your doctor won't decide. The committee will decide—when it meets." (Under the bill, the utilization committees were to be set up by the hospitals and be answerable to the hospitals—not the government, which was forbidden to interfere in any way. Many of the better hospitals in the country already had such committees, and Blue Cross had recommended making them mandatory for accreditation. Subsequently the Joint Board of Accreditation, of which the A.M.A. is a member, did make them mandatory.)

In conclusion, Dr. Annis addressed himself to "the millions of Americans who may have a doubt," and said, "I implore you as your doctor, ask your doctor."

27

"PRESIDENTS have tried to marshal public opinion before this for a favored and politically potent bill, but probably never on such a scale as has Mr. Kennedy for the health measure," the *Times* commented after the President's address in New York. Although Dr. Annis was generally credited with having won the contest in the Garden—as one union official put it, "his distortions were simply more credible than Kennedy's truths" —the whole experience seemed to have stiffened the President's determination to get the bill passed. For some time, he had been trying to bring several anti-Medicare men on the House Ways and Means Committee around and had persistently kept after its chairman to come out for the measure. Mills, who was described by Sorensen as being "tentatively opposed," finally sent word to the White House, through Speaker John McCormack, that he would do what he could, given enough time, and suggested that the best approach would be to attach Medicare as a rider in the Senate when a bill that had been passed in the House came up for a vote; that way, his committee would be circumvented, and the bill could emerge from the joint conference committee right onto the floor of the House. That strategy hadn't worked when it was tried in the special session of Congress just before the 1960 campaign, and the prospects didn't appear much better now. However, the 1960 defeat had produced an effective issue for the campaign that fall, and there was no reason to believe that if it had worked once, it wouldn't work again.

The administration waited to make a move until early July, when the Senate began debating a bill to implement President Kennedy's public-welfare program—a measure that the

House had already passed. The debate was perfunctory until Senator Anderson rose and offered Medicare as an amendment to the public-welfare bill. The A.M.A. had apparently been expecting the move. "The pressure was the most intense I've ever experienced," a senator from the West observed not long afterward. "I had made it absolutely clear that I was going to vote for the bill, but the A.M.A. wouldn't listen. They sent a delegation from home to visit me—my doctor, my wife's doctor, three other doctors I was friendly with back home, and four state party officials who had a lot to say about campaign funds. They were here for a week, and they pounded away at me every chance they got. It was intolerable. I learned later that the local medical society picked up the tab for their trip, which came to over five thousand dollars." Doctors from all over the country flew into Washington by the thousands—some of them in Senator Kerr's private plane, which he put at A.M.A.'s disposal. Medical societies in states near the capital visited their senators *en masse*, and doctors who were on vacation in the vicinity stopped off in Washington to make their views known.

On July 10th, Lawrence O'Brien, the chief White House liaison man with Congress, reported to the President that a head count in the Senate showed a lineup of fifty-one to forty-nine in favor of the bill, as a result of switches by four liberal Republicans and one moderate Southern Democrat from their 1960 positions. However, doubts were raised almost immediately about the head count; it had been made by Robert Baker, the secretary to the Senate majority, who enjoyed a far closer relationship with Kerr than with his boss, Senator Mike Mansfield, of Montana, the Majority Leader. A week later, O'Brien reported that he had made a head count of his own, which showed a fifty-fifty tie vote at best, and he added, "Senator Randolph has a problem." This was Jennings Randolph, Democrat of West Virginia, and his problem was that his state had spent more federal funds on various welfare programs than it was entitled to, and was faced with an unmanageable debt. Kerr gave him a way out—a clause in the public-welfare bill forgiving his state its indebtedness. It was assumed in the

147

White House that the favor expected from Randolph in return was his vote against Medicare, which he had backed in 1960.

President Kennedy, Democratic officials in West Virginia, and influential labor leaders went to work on Randolph to keep him in line. Before the final vote was taken, on July 17th, the administration was assured that forty-eight votes were solid for Medicare. In addition, Senator Carl Hayden, Democrat of Arizona, had told the administration that he could be counted on if his vote was needed to win, but that if it wasn't, he would cast it against Medicare. With Randolph and Hayden supporting the measure, the vote would have ended in a tie, which the Vice-President would have broken in favor of the bill. When a vote was taken on a motion to table the amendment, however, Randolph returned Kerr's favor. Hayden went along with Randolph, and the bill was defeated, fifty-two to forty-eight. President Kennedy, Sorensen wrote later, "never got over the disappointment of this defeat." The President went on television to tell the public that it had been a "most serious defeat for every American family," and then he ordered the Director of the Budget to cancel a public-works project for West Virginia.

The leaders of the A.M.A. were jubilant—to the point, apparently, where they began to feel that they had won not just another battle but the war itself. In large part, their confidence was based on a new Gallup poll, showing that public support for Medicare had fallen from sixty-seven per cent the year before to forty-four per cent. But Hutton and his National Council of Senior Citizens had by no means given up hope. In commenting on the vote in the Senate, he said, "The significant thing was that when two-thirds of the public supported the bill, back in 1960, it lost by seven votes. Now, with less than half the people supporting it, it lost by only one vote, discounting Hayden's. That made it clear that the Senate knew the people were being fooled, and didn't intend to be fooled much longer itself. And we all knew that the people wouldn't go on being fooled, either. All the publicity in the world won't convince a man that he isn't hungry when he *is* hungry."

As the law required, the national headquarters of AMPAC filed an affidavit with the government declaring its expenditures for the 1962 congressional campaign—$248,484. The figure did not include its outlays for "educational" purposes or any of the money spent by its state and county affiliates, which were not subject to federal law. According to Joe D. Miller, AMPAC's executive director, the national office handled only one out of every six dollars contributed by doctors; the remaining five were raised and spent locally, and were not reported. On the basis of this ratio, the nation's physicians put a million and a half dollars into some seventy House and a dozen Senate races. Representative King charged on the floor of the House that they had actually spent seven million dollars, and there were those who felt that even this figure was too low.

One rather sizable indirect contribution to the 1962 campaign came from the Blue Cross Association. Shortly before the election, it placed large advertisements in *Life, Newsweek,* the *Saturday Evening Post, Time,* and *Look* announcing once again that it was offering "amplified programs of protection" for the aged. Senator Harrison A. Williams, Democrat of New Jersey, instructed his staff to call Blue Cross offices around the country and check on the new plan; thirty-three offices were called, and not one of them had heard of it. The announcement, Williams said in the Senate, "was obviously politically motivated and a hoax on our older citizens." It was also questionable on another ground: the cost of the advertisements—in the neighborhood of a hundred thousand dollars—was paid by Blue Cross subscribers (since it came out of premiums paid in) and by the taxpayers (since Blue Cross, as a non-profit organization, is tax-exempt).

The results of organized medicine's participation in the congressional elections of 1962 were not impressive. In an average off-year election, the party in power loses thirty-nine seats in the House and two or three in the Senate. In that year's election, the Democrats lost two seats in the House and picked up four in the Senate. Not a single seat was lost by a candidate who had campaigned for Medicare. Doctors fought fiercely for Representative Walter Judd, Republican of Minnesota and a fellow-physician, but he was defeated. They fought fiercely against Senator Olin D. Johnston, Democrat of South Carolina, who had defected to the Medicare forces that year, but he won. In Miami, Dr. Annis's home town, the medical society waged one of the bitterest battles of the year against former Senator Claude Pepper, who was running for the House in an attempt at a comeback. In the late thirties and throughout the forties, Pepper had been one of the Senate's most outspoken advocates of national health insurance, and the A.M.A. had helped take his seat in the Senate away from him in 1950, when it successfully backed a former protégé of his, George Smathers, in the Democratic primary. In the 1962 Democratic primary, Pepper piled up a bigger vote than all three of his opponents, and went on to win the election in a walkaway.

"The A.M.A. committed political suicide in 1962," one veteran Washington reporter said after the election. "They went all out in supporting men who couldn't win and in opposing men who couldn't lose. They've never learned that just because you want something badly doesn't mean that you're going to get it."

The general failure of the A.M.A.'s ambitious venture into big-time national politics was not lost on Congress. Neither was a rather poignant demonstration of the fact that the medical profession was prepared to turn on even its oldest friends. The A.M.A. had always been able to count on the support of Senator Lister Hill, of Alabama, whose father, a doctor, had named him after Joseph Lister, the originator of the principle of antisepsis. Hill had been chiefly responsible for the Hill-Burton Act of 1946, which provided large federal funds for the construction and expansion of hospitals across the country. That law had created three hundred thousand additional hospital beds, along with two thousand clinics, laboratories, and diagnostic centers. The benefit to the nation's doctors was enormous since it created an enormous demand for medical services; moreover, the capital investment that automatically becomes available to a doctor when he gets hospital staff privileges is upwards of seventy thousand dollars—in this case, most of it coming from public funds. At any rate, in the 1962 vote on Medicare, Hill not only sided with the A.M.A. but persuaded his colleague from Alabama, Senator John Sparkman, to go along with him, thereby providing the winning margin. But Hill was a moderate in general, and when he came up for reëlection in 1962, Alabama doctors apparently decided that they did not care for moderation. After a bruising fight, which Hill won by the narrowest margin of his career, he was reported to be deeply embittered by the treatment he had received at the hands of his old friends, and it was predicted that he would not come to their aid again. The prediction proved to be correct. When Medicare was finally enacted Hill voted for it, and he persuaded Sparkman to go along with him.

One of the few races in 1962 that organized medicine may have won demonstrated to members of Congress that they couldn't protect themselves by remaining neutral, either. Representative Walter Moeller, a Democrat from Ohio, hadn't made up his mind about Medicare yet and refused to promise the doctors in his district that he would come out against the bill. That was enough to make them come out against him. "They made me a prime target," he recalled not long ago. "Dozens of doctors wrote and told me that they were going to work night and day to see that I was defeated. Their campaign was vicious—just vicious. They spread word that I was a Socialist, if not worse, and they even lectured their patients before treating them. One woman told me that her doctor threatened to stop taking care of her if she voted for me. Of course, they didn't say anything about my being a Lutheran pastor, or about my being one of the few members of the House who scrimps and saves on his office budget and turns the surplus back to the government. Anyway, their campaign seemed to have worked, although it's hard to say for sure, because 1962 was a bad year generally for Democrats in Ohio." The year 1964 was a better one for Moeller; he was elected to his old seat on a pro-Medicare platform.

Dr. Annis became president-elect of the A.M.A. in the summer of 1962, and shortly after the congressional elections that year, he addressed a meeting of the Public Relations Society of America and said that although the A.M.A.'s expenditures had been substantial, they had not been enough. "The siren songs of the politicians were more appealing than the voices of reason and experience," he declared. He went on to say that the medical profession would now have to step up its "educational campaign," especially through national advertising, but that, even so, it would be up to the individual doctor to carry most of the fight. "We want the whole truth, not the incomplete and distorted story, told, and the local physician, acting as a citizen, will be the one to do it," he explained. When someone mentioned the fact that many doctors avoided any kind of newspaper publicity, out of reluctance to do anything that might constitute unethical self-advertising, Dr. Annis advised reporters to get in touch with local medical societies if doctors refused to be quoted. "The sin of silence will no longer be condoned," he said.

28

ONE OF the A.M.A.'s persistent complaints about Medicare in 1962 was that it didn't cover the three million people sixty-five or over who were not in the Social Security program. When President Kennedy remedied this shortcoming early in 1963 by presenting a revised bill, which extended coverage to those three million, the A.M.A. condemned the new measure on the ground that it was "more sweeping" than its predecessor. The bill was put on the shelf that year, because the Ways and Means Committee, where all such legislation must originate, was fully occupied with consideration of an omnibus tax measure that the President considered to be of more immediate importance.

During the legislative lull, both sides in the Medicare battle concentrated on strengthening their support outside Washington. By this time, the National Council of Senior Citizens had over a million and a half members. The more active among them spoke at meetings of social clubs, distributed literature produced by the council, and continued a program of letter-writing to congressmen. As for the A.M.A., in March of 1963 it organized a plan called Operation Hometown, as part of a continuing effort to keep local medical societies involved —an effort that had received greater emphasis since the large turnout for AMPAC had suggested that doctors would give money in direct ratio to the control they retained over the way it was spent.

In order to "stimulate every voter to let his Congressman know that Medicare is really 'Fedicare'—a costly concoction of bureaucracy, bad medicine, and an unbalanced budget," the A.M.A. sent each local society a package containing seven thick folders of materials, with directions for using them. Among other things, there were speeches, from ten to twenty minutes long, accompanied by a "check list" that advised speakers to "look interested during the meeting," to "be friendly, warm, humble, *smile*," to "radiate authority," to "avoid scratching," and to "quit while you are ahead." There were several pamphlets, including one that was described as a "statement-sized pamphlet containing a personal message from doctor to patients," and some canned radio "interviews" in question-and-answer form, which were designed for medical or non-medical audiences. One of a number of booklets that were available for placement in doctors' offices, drugstores, and veterinarians' waiting rooms was entitled "New Concept of Aging," and it asserted that "there are no problems of people over sixty-five, except those imposed by retirement, that are not also the problems of all other age groups." To prove its case, the booklet cited the 1959 mortality tables, which showed that twenty-five children under the age of five had died of arteriosclerotic heart disease and that eight people over the age of sixty-five had died of infantile paralysis. "The term 'problems of aging,'" the booklet concluded, "is outmoded."

Advertising mats that the A.M.A. distributed in the course of Operation Hometown showed a gradual shift of emphasis that was clearly intended to win over the low-income workingman. "Can you afford a 16% increase in your payroll tax?" several of the advertisements asked. "That is the minimum payroll tax increase all workers earning $100 or more a week would be forced to pay if the Medicare bill now before Congress becomes law." This must have sounded to some people as if the total taxes taken out of their pay checks, including income taxes, would go up by sixteen per cent to pay for Medicare. Actually, the increase would affect only the Social Security tax, and, furthermore, the specific increase for Medicare would be not sixteen per cent but ten per cent. (The remaining six provided for in the bill was to pay for an increase in Social Security cash benefits.) The maximum increase would be less than eighteen dollars a year, with the average being about twelve dollars. In any event, the sixteen-per-cent figure apparently didn't sound bad enough, and it was later changed to twenty-three per cent. Since the maximum taxable wage base under the bill was $5,200, the A.M.A. was able to point out that a man making a hundred dollars a week would pay as much tax as a man making a hundred thousand dollars a year. This was true—and had always been —of the entire Social Security system.

Dr. Annis was especially fond of the suggestion that the poor would be paying for the medical care of the rich. "When I'm in Chicago riding in a taxi," he would tell groups of his colleagues, "I wait until I see an elderly couple in a Cadillac drive by, and then I ask the cabdriver if he wants to pay for their medical bills. 'No, sir,' says that cabdriver."

As its contribution to Operation Hometown, AMPAC sent out five thousand recordings of a talk that it claimed Paul Normile, a member of the executive board of the United Steelworkers, had given to some of his co-unionists. In the recording, a tough-sounding voice demanded that funds be collected for use in electing pro-Medicare candidates to Congress. "For those that don't want to give, you shop stewards can always let them know there is still a graveyard shift," the voice said at one point. "They'll kick in." AMPAC suggested that state and county medical societies use the recording "to stimulate membership dollars both for you and AMPAC." It at least stimulated Normile. He sued AMPAC for four hundred thousand dollars, charging that the recording was slanderous, because the voice was not his. At the trial, the executive director of the Pennsylvania branch of AMPAC testified that a man named Irv had told him that a man who called himself Cousin had an interesting record, and that he had met Cousin on a dark street corner one night and had bought the recording from him for twenty dollars. The A.M.A., assuming responsibility for the actions of its political affiliate, printed an apology to Normile in its *Journal,* and paid him twenty-five thousand dollars.

29

THE House Committee on Ways and Means completed its work on the tax bill late in the 1963 session, and convened in November for another round of hearings on government health insurance. A rather heated exchange took place on the fifth day, while Representative Al Ullman, Democrat of Oregon, was questioning H. Lewis Rietz, who was testifying as a representative of five hundred and twenty-five insurance companies—nine-tenths of the industry. Ullman was particularly interested in a claim by Rietz that fifty-three per cent of all people sixty-five and over were covered by voluntary health insurance—a claim that the A.M.A. was using in almost every advertisement it published (and that was later shown in a Senate investigation to be twice as high as the actual figure). After determining that the witness was unable to give any figures that would show what kind of coverage this insurance provided, Ullman said, "I am reminded of the story about the horse-rabbit stew that was advertised as half and half. When pinned down, it was one horse and one rabbit, so I think we should know what we are talking about when we discuss coverage. . . . Unless we know the quality of coverage, we know virtually nothing." Not long after that, the committee's chief counsel hurried into the room and whispered something to Chairman Mills. Turning pale, Mills interrupted the proceedings to announce that President Kennedy had been shot, and then adjourned the hearings.

At about the same moment, Henry Hall Wilson, a member of the White House congressional-liaison staff, left the Department of Health, Education and Welfare, where he had been discussing Mills's position on Medicare with Wilbur Cohen, whom President Kennedy had brought back into public life after five years of political exile at the University of Michigan. When the President appointed Cohen as H.E.W.'s Assistant Secretary for Legislation, Senator Smathers, at the request of the A.M.A., tried to block the appointment in the Senate—until the President warned Smathers to leave Cohen alone. Now, as a secretary rushed in to tell him about the assassination, Cohen was going over a memorandum that he and Wilson had drawn up, at the President's request, outlining several ways that Mills's objections to the Medicare bill might be met. After the news of the President's death was confirmed, Cohen, like millions of other people, went home to be with his family, and spent most of the next few days sitting, dazed, before his television screen. The following Monday, an hour or so after the funeral, Wilson telephoned him at home and told him that O'Brien thought President Johnson should see the memorandum they had been working on. Cohen and his wife drove to his office, his wife typed up the memorandum, and they took it over to the White House. Members of the staff were milling about more or less aimlessly, and Cohen made his way through them to Sorensen's office. "He was there alone, a numbed pallor on his face," Cohen recalled afterward. Leaving the office quietly, Cohen took the memorandum to Wilson, who said that he would show it to the President.

Mr. Johnson's views on many matters were unknown when he succeeded to the Presidency, but he was clearly on record as supporting Medicare. "Why anyone would want to deny a person the opportunity of putting in a dollar a month, along with his employer, to insure himself through Social Security against the staggering costs of hospitalization simply amazes me," he had said to the executive board of the National Council of Senior Citizens the previous summer. In his first address to a joint session of Congress after assuming office, he called for action on "the dream of health care for the elderly." According to *Medical Economics*, "the Medicare program's chances have never been better." President Johnson was asked about its chances at one of his early press conferences, and he replied that he thought Congress would act sometime in 1964. He added, "I can think of no piece of legislation that I would be happier to approve than that bill."

30

LOGROLLING is as much a part of politics as it is of lumbering —and is often as hazardous. Over the years, the A.M.A. had made alliances with various organizations that agreed to support it in its fight against government health insurance. In such arrangements, there usually comes a time when the favor has to be returned. In March of 1963, the A.M.A. announced that it was discontinuing a study of the physiological effects of smoking, because the Surgeon General had undertaken a thorough examination of the problem, but the following December the Association suddenly decided to go ahead with its study. Early in January, 1964, shortly before the Surgeon General issued his report on smoking, Dr. Annis, speaking before the Kentucky legislature, warned its members that the forthcoming government report would undoubtedly present "insurmountable evidence that smoking causes cancer." He added that "the A.M.A. is not opposed to smoking and tobacco, but it is opposed to disease," and then he launched into an attack on Medicare. "The choice of these two topics in a tobacco-state address was just pure coincidence, of course," Representative Frank Thompson, Democrat of New Jersey, remarked at the time.

The Surgeon General's report was made public on January 11th, and as Dr. Annis had predicted, it unequivocally attributed various forms of cancer to cigarette smoking. Afterward, Representative Harold D. Cooley, of North Carolina, who was chairman of the House Agriculture Committee, called for a crash research program to discover what ingredient in tobacco was doing the damage and to find some way of eliminating it. Cigarette manufacturers appeared unwilling to concede that any damage was being done. So did the A.M.A. On February 7th, the A.M.A. announced that six leading cigarette companies had granted it a total of ten million dollars to set up a tobacco-research institute for the purpose of studying the problem—if, indeed, there was a problem. "The A.M.A. has made a deal with the tobacco industry . . . to get tobacco-state congressmen to vote against Medicare," Thompson charged. "It's an outrage." When the Association objected to what it called "an unjustified assault on the integrity" of its officers, Thompson replied that the behavior of the A.M.A. itself was "an assault on the faith Americans have traditionally placed in their doctors." In effect, he went on, the A.M.A. was encouraging people "to ignore the proven dangers of tobacco and to continue smoking."

Not long afterward, the Federal Trade Commission ordered that cigarette packages and cigarette advertisements carry a warning about the hazards of smoking. The A.M.A. opposed the order, because, it said, everyone already knew the dangers of smoking. "More than 90 million persons in the United States use tobacco in some form," the A.M.A. stated in a letter of protest to the commission. "Long-standing social customs and practices are established in the use of tobacco; the economic lives of tobacco growers, processers, and merchants are entwined in the industry; and local, state, and the federal governments are the recipients of and dependent upon many millions of dollars of tax revenue." Senator Maurine Neuberger, Democrat of Oregon, rose on the floor of the Senate to comment on the A.M.A.'s new tobacco-research institute and on the letter to the F.T.C. "I have no way of knowing whether or not the statement by the A.M.A. to the Federal Trade Commission represents the first fruits of this extensive research program," she said. In any event, she went on, "I find myself growing somewhat apprehensive about the concern of the A.M.A. for the economic well-being of the tobacco industry rather than the physical well-being of smokers or potential smokers."

Many doctors around the country shared her apprehension. The *Medical Tribune* reported that according to a recent survey ninety-five per cent of the country's physicians thought smoking was harmful. Some of them, dismayed at the stand that their official representatives had taken, registered objections with the A.M.A.'s national office and with their local medical societies. "We were no less than flabbergasted," a generally conservative medical journal called *GP* commented editorially on the A.M.A.'s refusal to endorse the Surgeon General's report. It added that it would like to see, for once, "a little more integrity and a lot less squirming."

Since it was necessary for the A.M.A. to respond to the outcry in some fashion, it published a folder called "Smoking: Facts You Should Know." At the beginning, the text pointed out that there were "hidden costs of smoking," among which were the price of cigarettes, forest fires, marred furniture, and holes in rugs and clothing. Next, the folder brought up "suspected health hazards," and listed the afflictions that smoking was "alleged to cause." The conclusion, in which not even a congressman from a tobacco-growing state could find much to take offense at, was:

> Physicians and researchers who believe these observations to be correct, say, "Don't smoke! If you do smoke, quit. If you don't smoke, don't start." Some equally competent physicians and research personnel are less sure of the effect of cigarette smoking on health. They believe the increase in these diseases can be explained by other factors in our complex environment. They advise, "Smoke if you feel you should, but be moderate."

31

On March 25, 1964, the *Wall Street Journal* predicted that Medicare was "a good bet to come out of Congress this year." People in the White House were not so sure. The main obstacle was still the House Ways and Means Committee, and the only certainty about the lineup of its members was that it was unfavorable—either fourteen to eleven against the bill or thirteen to twelve against it. There were ten Republicans on the committee, all of them opposed, and at least three of the fifteen Democrats were also opposed: Mills; A. Sydney Herlong, of Florida; and John C. Watts, of Kentucky. The doubtful member was Clark W. Thompson, of Texas, who had formerly opposed the bill but now wouldn't say where he stood. Late that winter, *Congressional Quarterly*, which is read very carefully in Washington, published an "exclusive" report to the effect that Mills was now convinced that the Kerr-Mills program had failed, and was about to capitulate. The A.M.A. immediately sent one of its lobbyists over to Capitol Hill to get a public denial from Mills. Although he was upset by the story, which he believed had been planted by someone in the administration to put him on the spot, Mills refused to deny it, thus adding to the uncertainty.

In April, after more public hearings on Medicare, the Ways and Means Committee went into executive session. "Prospects of favorable action are no better and perhaps a bit worse than they've been from the start," a member of the committee told a reporter. President Johnson seized every opportunity to improve the prospects. After some high officials of the United States Chamber of Commerce, which still opposed even the Kerr-Mills program, had a meeting with the President at the

White House, one of the participants declared him to have been "almost a zealot" in presenting the case for Medicare. Citing as an example an elderly, bedridden man on public welfare, Mr. Johnson reminded the businessmen that welfare was paid for out of tax funds. Not bothering to remind them who paid the highest taxes, he went on to point out that if Medicare had been in effect during the man's working life, the money contributed from his wages to the Social Security fund would have provided a lump sum of four thousand dollars to pay for his care, thereby reducing the need for welfare aid, and reducing taxes as well. Several of his listeners were converted then and there. Representative Clark Thompson was also converted, after a reminder that the President had written to twenty-five hundred of Thompson's constituents during his last primary fight back home in Texas. The lineup on the Ways and Means Committee was now thirteen to twelve against the bill.

Early that summer, it suddenly looked as if the balance had become fourteen to eleven in favor of the bill. Mills reported to the administration that Representative Watts had said he was ready to switch, and had gone as far as to give Mills his proxy. This change, Mills added, made it possible for him to support Medicare, too. Explaining that he hadn't wanted his own vote to be the decisive one, and thus bring down on his head the wrath of the medical profession, he said that once Watts had changed over, making it thirteen to twelve for the bill, he felt he could go along. It would be a simple matter, he said, to justify his move to the doctors by pointing out to them that in this way he would retain control over the measure and could stop it from becoming any less acceptable to them than it already was. But then, on June 23rd, the day before the committee was due to take a vote, Watts took back his proxy and told Mills that he intended to oppose the bill. When King learned that Watts had backed down, he withdrew his request for a vote on the bill, to avoid having an adverse vote entered in the record. "The alliance between the tobacco industry and the American Medical Association caused the defeat of the Medicare program in the House Ways and Means Committee," William V. Shannon wrote in his column in the New York *Post*. "Watts represents a district in western Kentucky in which tobacco is the principal crop."

In earlier deliberations, the committee had approved a five-per-cent increase in Social Security benefits, the first since 1958. Now the ranking Republican on the committee, John W. Byrnes, of Wisconsin, made what struck his colleagues as an unexpected and un-Republican move: he proposed that the increase be six per cent instead. To pay for the five-per-cent increase, the committee had already decided to raise the total tax imposed on both employers and employees to just under nine and a half per cent. It had been widely accepted in Congress that the Social Security tax should never go above ten per cent, and Ullman saw that Byrnes's aim was to bring the rate above nine and a half per cent by means of the six-per-cent increase, and so leave no room for the one-half of one per cent required to pay for Medicare. He quickly explained this to the other members of the committee who favored Medicare, and urged them to stand fast. One liberal Democrat was absent, which meant that twenty-four members were on hand for the roll call. All the Democrats except Mills, Herlong, and Watts stuck by Ullman, giving his side eleven votes. Eight Republicans voted with Byrnes, and they were joined by the three conservative Democrats who opposed Medicare, giving the proposal twelve votes. The Medicare supporters were in despair, for the one vote still to be cast was that of Bruce Alger, an arch-conservative Republican from Dallas. Everyone was dumbfounded when Alger voted against the six-per-cent increase, making it a twelve-to-twelve standoff, which defeated the proposal. Afterward, Alger explained that since he opposed the entire Social Security system, consistency would not permit him to vote to expand it.

After that, Social Security amendments based on a five-per-cent increase were reported out by the Ways and Means Committee, and approved by the House with only eight negative votes. Nearly all congressmen wanted to be able to claim some credit at election time for giving their elderly constituents at least a little financial assistance. The administration

164

was said to be planning to attach Medicare to the House Social Security bill when it came up in the Senate, but it was generally agreed that, as the *Wall Street Journal* put it at the time, "if it appears at any stage that the Medicare issue would kill the Social Security measure, the Medicare campaign would be allowed to collapse so that a cash-benefits-increasing measure could be rushed to President Johnson before adjournment."

Congress recessed briefly in July for the Republican National Convention and again in August for the Democratic National Convention, and then reconvened to dispose of the final business of the session—a food-stamp program for the needy, a housing bill, and the Social Security amendments. In the Senate, the last of these were the responsibility of the Finance Committee, which revised the amendments and passed them on to the floor without any provision for Medicare. Before anyone had a chance to attach the King-Anderson bill as a rider, Senator Russell Long, of Louisiana, went Congressman Byrnes one better by proposing that the cash increase be seven per cent. Senator Albert Gore, of Tennessee, jumped to his feet. "The effect of this amendment would be to kill Medicare forever," he said. ("Well, that's the idea," Smathers remarked to a reporter afterward.)

Long had always disapproved of Medicare. Besides having influential friends in the medical profession and the insurance industry, he had political motives that no one would have understood better than his father, the late Huey P. Long. "Like his father, Russell wants every man to be a king," one senator has said. "And, like his father, he, and he alone, is going to be the one who passes out the crowns. The Long family's lexicon simply doesn't include the term 'social insurance' —that is, making somebody relatively independent by taking money from him when he is working and healthy and then giving it back to him when he retires or is out of a job or gets sick. Russell doesn't comprehend that concept. Federal money to be distributed in Louisiana through the Long machine is one thing, but federal money that goes directly to his constituents is quite another. Just consider the effect if several hundred thousand old people who hadn't been able to get medical care without welfare assistance, courtesy of the Longs, suddenly found that they could get it without going on the dole—and without having to thank anyone!"

During the Senate debate on Long's proposal, which was eventually defeated, Gore taunted him about the amount of the help he was prepared to give the common man—pension increases ranging from ninety cents to two dollars and fifty-four cents a month—compared to the relief from burdensome and often insupportable medical expenses which he was working against. But Gore was less interested in arguing with Long than in holding off a vote until other senators could prepare a suitable version of Medicare in the form of an amendment. When it was ready, Gore still had the floor, and he presented the amendment for a vote. Four liberal Republicans had let it be known that they were coming over to the administration's side, so everyone assumed that the amendment would win—except Senator Goldwater, who was under the impression that he held the swing vote, and flew back from Arizona on September 2nd to cast it against Medicare. For a while, it looked as if his estimate were correct, since the tally stood at forty-two to forty-two, but then some more senators arrived and made it forty-nine to forty-four in favor. It was the first time that any health-insurance legislation had been passed in either house.

32

ALTHOUGH the Senate's action was unsettling to the leaders of the A.M.A., they appeared to be confident that their friends would look after their interests when the joint conference committee met to adjust the differences between the House and Senate bills. Their confidence appeared to be justified. Of the Senate conferees—seven of them, chosen on the basis of committee seniority—only Gore and Anderson supported Medicare. The other Democrats were Long, Smathers, and the chairman of the Finance Committee, Harry Flood Byrd, of Virginia. The Republicans were John J. Williams, of Delaware, and Frank Carlson, of Kansas. Of the House conferees, who numbered five, only two were in favor of the bill—King, its co-sponsor, and Hale Boggs, of Louisiana, the Majority Whip. Mills, who was the chairman of the conference committee, and the two Republicans from the House—Byrnes and Thomas Curtis, of Missouri—were opposed.

By tradition, conferees function as blocs, and each bloc is expected to defend the position of the body it represents. Since the House had not voted on Medicare, Mills was relatively free to interpret things as he wanted to, but the vote in the Senate required Byrd and the other senators to stand by Medicare—up to a point. Also by tradition, the determination of where that point lies is made by the conferees; while it is true that if they ignore the wishes of the body they represent, as expressed in its vote, it may repudiate their action by rejecting the conference report, the report is almost always approved as a matter of course in a final vote in each house.

During the conference committee's deliberations, which dragged on for nearly a month that fall, Mills repeatedly indicated that he was willing to come to terms with the Medicare people, they repeatedly offered compromises of one kind or another, and he repeatedly discussed them at great length and then turned them down. After a couple of weeks of this, Anderson, Gore, King, and Boggs had become so desperate that they were willing to take practically anything that would get Medicare started. "We were ready to accept ten days of hospitalization and nothing else," one of them said afterward. Putting on a brave front, they offered Mills a compromise: if he would give them forty-five days of hospital coverage, they would give up the other sections of the bill. Mills thought it over, and said that he would accept the offer. But when they presented it in writing, he raised a complicated procedural objection and postponed a vote.

After that session, one of the participants sent a note to the President that said, in part, "Mills appeared to believe he had the conferees boxed in where they would have to accept the Social Security benefits increase without Medicare. I believe that Mills does not think the Medicare conferees or the administration will have the courage to object to a benefits-increase bill by itself." The note also informed the President that if the cash increase should be permitted to go through without any health-insurance provisions, it might well be impossible to persuade Congress to raise Social Security taxes again the following year to pay for Medicare. Partly as a result of this appraisal, Boggs flatly warned Mills at the next meeting of the committee that he might refuse to sign the conference report if it didn't include some form of Medicare. Mills, the chairman of one of the most powerful committees on the Hill, was clearly taken aback by this, for Boggs, as Majority Whip, had a fair amount of power of his own, and throughout his political career Mills had always sought to avoid the sort of collision that Boggs was threatening to bring about. Then Gore and Anderson told Mills that they would ask the Senate to reject the conference report unless there was at least a compromise on Medicare. Faced with these unprecedented threats to his standing in Congress, Mills reluctantly agreed to consider the compromise, and asked that it be drafted as a com-

168

pleted amendment, so that the committee could go over it the following week.

As the meeting broke up, one of the conferees remarked to a colleague that he had misjudged Mills. "Before, I wondered whether he was completely lacking in integrity," he said. "Now I know." In politics, "integrity" has a looser meaning than it has in most other lines of work—a distinction that is perhaps best illustrated by the old Washington saw that a statesman is a politician who stays bought. Be that as it may, nearly everyone in Washington has always considered Mills a man of integrity. The slighting remark, made in the heat of the moment, did not take fully into account the complexity of the predicament facing Mills. Although the reports that he had given certain assurances to friends in medical circles undoubtedly had substance, a more compelling reason for his intransigence on Medicare was that, as overseer in the House of the Social Security system, he was seriously concerned about keeping it soundly financed, and feared that something like Medicare would sooner or later put it out of balance.

Another reason was that he believed there were not enough votes in the House to assure passage of the bill. As chairman of the Ways and Means Committee, he was unwilling to take a bill to the floor if it seemed likely to be beaten. That had happened in 1958, with the first measure he had taken to the floor as chairman of the committee, and he had not forgotten the shock. (By tradition, bills coming out of the Ways and Means Committee are given a "closed rule" by the Rules Committee, which means that they are not subject to the usual amending process on the floor. Nearly all bills presented by the committee's chairman are either voted up or voted down, and because of the lack of debate, and of the general confusion that ordinarily attends the voting, success or failure is invariably laid to the chairman.)

Still another reason for Mills's reluctance was that roughly three-quarters of the members of the House didn't want to vote that year on Medicare, regardless of their feelings about it. Scores of them, on both sides of the aisle and from both the pro-Medicare and the anti-Medicare camps, had privately appealed to Mills to block the bill in committee. "They didn't want to go home just before the election and face the big campaign spenders—the medical societies, the chambers of commerce, the insurance industry—who would be sure to get them if they voted for Medicare," one member of the committee who had discussed the problem with Mills remarked later. "And if they voted *against* Medicare, the old folks and the unions would go after them." Any committee chairman would be sensitive to this kind of appeal, the congressman added, because if he kept his friends out of trouble by taking the blame himself, he could count on their gratitude—and on their support when he needed it.

Late that summer, Mills probably felt quite safe in the position he had taken, for the word from Arkansas was that Goldwater would sweep the state. By the end of September, though, it appeared that Republican sentiment had fallen off sharply and that Johnson would carry Arkansas. On September 28th—shortly before the conference committee went back into session to consider the compromise amendment—Mills got up before a luncheon meeting of the Kiwanis Club in Little Rock and hedged his bet. Denying that he had been responsible for blocking Medicare, as most newspapers claimed, he said, "I want to make it clear that I have always thought there was great appeal in the argument that wage earners, during their working lifetime, should make payments into a fund to guard against the risk of financial disaster due to heavy medical costs [after they retire]. . . . I am acutely aware of the fact that there is a problem here which must be met."

On October 2nd, when the conference committee convened to vote on the compromise amendment, Mills made it clear that he was not ready to meet the problem just then. Instead of approving the amendment, as he had led its proponents to believe he would, he called for a vote on the cash-increase amendments without Medicare. The two Republican conferees on the House side immediately sided with him, making the vote in the House bloc three to two, the minority being King and Boggs. After that, the two Republican senators abandoned the Senate's position to vote for the motion. Byrd, who apparently did not want to offend either the Senate or Mills, abstained for the moment. Then Gore and Anderson voted against the motion, making it a two-to-two standoff in the Senate bloc. Appearing quite confident of the remaining Senate votes, Mills called on Long. Long voted against him. Obviously astonished by this development, Mills turned to Smathers, who had never been known to let the A.M.A. down during almost twenty years in Congress. With his vote, and a vote from Byrd, who everyone assumed could be counted on to stand and deliver if the conservative cause was in danger, the motion would carry. After a pause, Smathers voted against the motion. Mills, ordinarily an impassive man, stared at him openmouthed. "He just couldn't believe that George had done it," one of the conferees said afterward. When Mills finally did come to believe it, he announced that the conference was deadlocked, and adjourned without reporting out any bill at all. As all the conferees knew when they left the room, they had created one of the big—perhaps the biggest— issues of the forthcoming Presidential and congressional campaigns. "It looks like the people will have to vote on Medicare," Senator Anderson said at the time.

The A.M.A. was as much surprised as Mills at the stand taken by Smathers and Long, and a good deal angrier. The Association's political tacticians had done everything they could think of to keep the two men in line, exerting constant pressure through their Washington lobbyists, arranging for incessant telephone calls from influential constituents, and seeing to it that they got bales of letters and telegrams from doctors back home. The Medicare group's methods were more compelling. Long wanted to be Majority Whip if Hubert Humphrey, the incumbent whip, was elected Vice-President, and in order to get the post he had to demonstrate that he was a loyal administration man. In addition, he had to win the approval of enough of his fellow-Democrats to be elected to the job. In exchange for Long's promise that he would hold to the Senate's position in the conference, Anderson had agreed to give Long his vote for whip, plus several other votes he controlled. As for Smathers, his explanation of why he had voted against Mills was simpler. "Lyndon told me to," he said.

Shortly after the Republican National Convention, a Doctors for Goldwater Committee was set up, with a roster of officers that the *New Republic* described as "a Who's Who of the American Medical Association." The committee's first appeal to the members of the A.M.A. brought in donations amounting to a hundred and fifty thousand dollars. At about the time this appeal went out, AMPAC declared that it would spend half a million dollars on selected House and Senate contests, and that its state affiliates were scheduled to spend five or six times that amount. Everyone in the so-called "medical family" was expected to help out. For instance, the Maryland Medical Political Action Committee sent letters to the wives of all doctors and dentists in the state asking for donations of ten dollars or more in addition to what their husbands were contributing. "Would you invest $10.00 to insure your children and grandchildren freedom under the Constitution as we have known it?" the letters asked.

It has been estimated that as many as a third of the members of the A.M.A.'s House of Delegates are also members of the John Birch Society. The letters sent out by the Maryland Medical Political Action Committee led to speculation about whether the Society had not at least had some influence among doctors in Maryland. After appealing for funds, the letters went on:

Dimitry Manuilsky, Soviet official, one-time presiding officer of the UN Security Council, said to the Lenin School of Political Warfare, Moscow, in 1930: "War to the hilt between Communism and Capitalism is inevitable. Today, of course, we are not strong enough to attack. Our time will come in 20 or 30 years. To win, we shall need the element of surprise. The bourgeoisie will have to be put to sleep. So we shall begin by launching the most spectacular peace movement on record. There will be electrifying overtures and unheard-of concessions. The Capitalist countries, stupid and decadent, will rejoice in their own destruction. They will leap at another chance

172

to be friends. As soon as their guard is down, we shall smash them with our clenched fist."

One woman who received this letter, the wife of a staff physician at Johns Hopkins, later reported that she asked a member of the committee what Manuilsky's statement had to do with Medicare, and whether the unheard-of concessions included the Berlin Wall and the Russian missile installations in Cuba. She got no answer.

Besides trying to influence members of Congress through campaign funds, organized medicine demonstrated its faith in the democratic process by trying to influence them through their constituents. Early in October, the A.M.A. unveiled a million-dollar advertising campaign, which it described as "a national education program to inform the public on the broad range of health care now available to the elderly." Although the campaign was to be conducted just before the elections, the A.M.A. declared that it was in no way intended to be political in nature. Its purpose, the Association stated, was "to highlight Community Health Week, October 18-24." In order to stress the importance of Community Health Week, the A.M.A. planned to run quarter-page advertisements in more than seven thousand weekly newspapers, full-page advertisements in daily newspapers in all cities with populations over a hundred thousand, and special full-page spreads in *Life*, the *Saturday Evening Post, Look, Newsweek, U.S. News & World Report*, and the *Saturday Review*. In addition, there were to be thirty one-minute TV spots for nationwide audiences and several hundred on local stations. Even the nation's clergymen were called on for help. Each of them received a "ministerial announcement" for inclusion in his services: "It would be well that during this Community Health Week we join in prayer in appreciation of the health services provided by the dedicated teams of physicians, nurses, technologists, and all workers who serve our community."

One of the advertisements that appeared in newspapers around the country stated, "A health program is available in

173

your community now that provides to every elderly person who needs it the health care he or she requires. We call this health program Health Opportunity Program for the Elderly." Everyone else called it the Kerr-Mills program. James R. Dumpson, the New York City Commissioner of Welfare, wrote to the New York State Medical Society to complain about "the questionable ethics" of this statement, which, he said, was clearly meant to convey the idea that the state had a new program—in addition to its Kerr-Mills program—to take care of the health needs of the elderly. His impression, he wrote, was "confirmed by a barrage of telephone calls to the New York City Department of Welfare by . . . residents who had been wholly misled by this advertisement." Elsewhere, people must have been even more confused, for the same advertisement appeared in twelve states where no Kerr-Mills programs existed.

Goldwater was not the only foe of Medicare to be defeated on November 3, 1964. Eleven of fourteen doctors who ran for Congress lost. One of the three who won supported Medicare; of the other two doctors, one was a long-time incumbent, and one ran in a safe district against a woman who was given little chance. Of more immediate significance, though, was the fact that the A.M.A. lost three of its most dependable allies on the Ways and Means Committee. In all, the pro-Medicare forces were strengthened by the addition of four votes in the Senate and forty-four votes in the House. An analysis of the election returns showed that twenty-two per cent of the vote had been cast by people over the age of sixty, two million of whom had switched from the Republican column to the Democratic. And though seven of the ten states with the highest percentage of elderly voters were traditionally Republican, all ten went to the Democrats.

Shortly after the election, Mills made another speech in Little Rock—this time before the Lions Club—in which he said, "I can support a payroll tax for financing health benefits just as I have supported a payroll tax for cash benefits." Speaker McCormack announced that Medicare would be the first order of business in the Eighty-ninth Congress. Mills announced

174

that he would be happy to present the bill to the Ways and Means Committee if the President asked him to. And the President announced that he would ask him to.

An A.M.A. convention was held in Miami late in November, and Dr. Donovan Ward, who had succeeded Dr. Annis as the Association's president, told the delegates that they had to "face up to certain grim realities," one of which was a "significant loss of votes" in Congress. But he went on to deride the notion that this meant that Medicare was certain to be enacted. Ordinarily, A.M.A. members are a tractable audience, but as the convention wore on, some of them began to grumble about the way the Association was spending their money. Finally, one of them got up and asked about a rumor he had heard to the effect that the publicity for Community Health Week had cost twice the one million dollars that the A.M.A.'s leaders had said it would. The trustees refused to confirm or deny the report. Disaffection took other forms, too. One member who appeared before the committee that was responsible for dealing with matters like Medicare—the Committee on Legislation and Public Relations—said, "The problem is not what to do but how you do it. And you're going to do it the way the people of the United States want you to." Another delegate urged the same committee to accept the fact that members of Congress were "not men of sinister purpose but men of high ideals." Then he added, "The public which has sent them to Congress has indicated it wants a positive approach to the problem of medical care for the aged—now."

Remarks like these had rarely been made at A.M.A. meetings. The delegations from Michigan and the District of Columbia went even further and proposed that the A.M.A. support at least a minimal role for the government in taking care of the aged. "We do not, by profession, compromise in matters of life and death," Dr. Ward reminded them sternly. "Nor can we compromise with honor and duty." The Michigan and District of Columbia proposals were defeated, but a proposal empowering the trustees to launch "an expanded educational effort during the next few months" was quickly approved. When a reporter asked a delegate why it was necessary to give the trustees authority they already had, he was told, "They seek a broad base to shoulder the criticism which will soon be heard against the waste of millions of dollars in lost political causes." No one seemed sure how much the effort to head off disaster in 1965 would cost, but one trustee was heard to remark that it would probably come to at least three and a half million dollars. The end was in sight, but the A.M.A. had not yet given up hope. At the close of the meeting, Dr. James Z. Appel, who was due to take over the presidency in June, said, "We'll use every gimmick we can."

33

ALTHOUGH a politician who has won an election invariably announces that he has been given a mandate to carry out all the campaign promises he made, it is usually impossible to determine whether the voters' support means that they share all, many, or even some of his views. Maybe they simply couldn't stand the other fellow. During the campaign of 1964, President Johnson made a great many promises, but he made none as often or as fervently as the promise that if he was elected he would see to it that Congress enacted the Medicare program. The supporters of the bill naturally interpreted Mr. Johnson's overwhelming victory at the polls as a complete triumph for their own cause. "Clearest Mandate for Medicare in Lyndon B. Johnson's Landslide," ran a headline in the *Senior Citizens News*, the monthly newsletter of the National Council of Senior Citizens, whose membership had by now risen to two and a half million. And, just as naturally, the American Medical Association dismissed claims of this sort out of hand. According to Dr. Ward, such statements constituted "an arrogant affront to the dignity and integrity of those who have just been elected." Those who had just been elected to Congress were far less impressed by all the claims and counterclaims about mandates than they were by the fact that most of the sixty-nine freshmen Democrats who had just been elected to the House of Representatives owed, or believed they owed, their victories to the Johnson landslide. Beyond that, a fair number of incumbents who occupied shaky seats were indebted to Mr. Johnson for help during the campaign. Accordingly, as far as most of the Democrats in the

House were concerned, if the President said he had a mandate for Medicare, he had a mandate for Medicare.

When President Johnson delivered his State of the Union Address on January 4, 1965, the first day of the Eighty-ninth Congress, and called for action on a Medicare bill as the first order of business, no one in the government doubted that he would get it. In a ceremonious response to his appeal, the Democratic leaders in Congress immediately arranged to let Senator Anderson and Representative King introduce identical bills, numbered S. 1 and H.R. 1, in the Senate and in the House. In its provisions for hospital and nursing-home care, the measure was much the same as one that Anderson and King had submitted to the previous Congress, but there was one significant change in its financing. Although Mills had come around to accepting the fact that some sort of Medicare bill was inevitable, he insisted upon protecting the actuarial soundness of the Social Security program by keeping the Medicare funds entirely separate from the program's pension funds, and the administration had acceded to his demand.

On the second day of Congress, the membership of the Ways and Means Committee, reflecting the Democrats' new majority in the House, of better than two to one, was changed from fifteen Democrats and ten Republicans to seventeen Democrats and eight Republicans. This gave the bill's supporters a margin of at least three votes on the committee, thus assuring that the measure would not be blocked there again. Moreover, there was a general feeling that the increase in Democratic support for Medicare had been attended by a lessening of Republican opposition. Polls showed that two-thirds of the nation's voters favored the bill, and it was believed that many Republicans were far more sensitive to public opinion on this topic than they had been a few months before. At the beginning of the session, Representative Frank T. Bow, a conservative Republican from Ohio, sent all members of his party in the House a letter in which he said in part, "Social Security and medical care were primary issues in 1964, and the Republican response on these issues was a major factor in the disaster that befell us." Representative Charles Halleck, of Indiana, who had played a large role in that disaster, was replaced as Minority Leader in the House by Representative Gerald Ford, of Michigan, who promised a program of positive opposition to the Democrats. Rumor had it that one move in this direction would be a Republican alternative to Medicare.

On January 7th, the President sent a special Health Message to Congress, in which he again called for passage of the King-Anderson bill. Afterward, Mills told reporters that he hoped to get it through his committee and onto the floor of the House by March. Despite Mills's earlier public statements to the effect that he was no longer opposed to Medicare, the A.M.A.'s leaders were stunned by this remark. "They were furious at Mills for what they considered the ultimate in perfidy," Michael J. O'Neill, a Washington correspondent for the New York *Daily News* who had covered A.M.A. activities for many years, said at the time. "And Mills was furious at them for their blind refusal to accept reality. They couldn't understand that on a great controversial issue like this one Mills wasn't a conservative or a liberal or a moderate. He was a politician. And he has always been a consummately adroit one. If he couldn't stop the bill, he was naturally going to turn it to his own purposes, even if it meant that he ended up sponsoring it."

A couple of days after Mills predicted prompt action on Medicare, about two hundred representatives of state medical societies met in Chicago, in accordance with arrangements that the A.M.A. had made the previous November. At the Chicago meeting, the Association's trustees reaffirmed their determination to fight on, and said they hoped to get Mills to reverse himself, or, failing that, to get the pro-Medicare people who had been elected to the House to reverse themselves. Several of those present pointed out that Mills, having finally put himself on record, could not possibly retreat, even if he wanted to. Moreover, they noted, if the new pro-Medicare margin in the House was cut by half—which was more than

179

anyone could reasonably hope—it would still be large enough to put the bill through. "To concede defeat is to invite it," one of the trustees told the rebels sternly.

In a surprise move, the trustees then informed the gathering that they had devised a new program, which, they stated, "would provide far more to our elderly citizens than is proposed in the administration's Medicare tax program." As the plan was outlined in broad terms by Dr. Ward, it would provide federal and state grants, under the provisions of the Kerr-Mills program, to subsidize private health-insurance policies for old people who wanted them. The A.M.A. called its plan the Doctors' Eldercare Program, and Dr. Ward announced that in order to secure support for Eldercare among doctors—whose enthusiasm for the expenditure of their own money was beginning to wane noticeably—and to arrange for still another publicity drive to arouse the lay public, the House of Delegates would meet early in February for a two-day special session.

On January 27th, the day the Ways and Means Committee convened to hold executive-session hearings on the King-Anderson bill, two of the A.M.A.'s closest friends on the committee—A. Sydney Herlong, Democrat of Florida, and Thomas B. Curtis, Republican of Missouri—introduced Eldercare in the House. Dr. Ward called the event a "breakthrough of historic importance." Apart from its sponsors, no one in Congress took the breakthrough very seriously. "Everyone in the House knows that it's nonsense," Representative Al Ullman, Democrat of Oregon, who was a leading Medicare supporter on the committee, said at the time. "By itself, it would provide little that cannot be done under existing law—that is, if the states agree to do it." He went on to suggest that since few states had been able to participate in the Kerr-Mills program to any appreciable extent, even fewer would be able to participate in the A.M.A.'s far more expensive plan through the same procedures. If all the states did participate, it was estimated, the program would cost them and the federal government a total of something like four billion dollars annually. Representative Frank Thompson, who had jousted with the A.M.A. over the

Surgeon General's report on smoking, expressed his opinion of Eldercare by suggesting an alternative to it, which he called Doctorcare. It was to be financed by a two-per-cent federal tax on applesauce, and the funds were to be used to provide special therapy for any physician who felt himself suffering from an urge to make house calls; if he didn't respond satisfactorily to the arguments of his colleagues over the phone, he was to be rushed to the nearest Cadillac showroom.

The day after Eldercare was dropped into the legislative hopper, Representative Byrnes, the ranking Republican on the Ways and Means Committee, announced that he had prepared a new bill that would pay just about every kind of medical expense incurred by the elderly. As one of the leading Republicans in the House, Byrnes was understood to be acting on a suggestion made by Minority Leader Ford. The Byrnes bill, which had actually been prepared by a leading insurance company, provided, like Eldercare, for subsidies to pay for private health-insurance policies. Unlike Eldercare, the disposition of the subsidies was to be in the hands of the federal government rather than of state governments—an arrangement that had always been unacceptable to the A.M.A. Two-thirds of the cost—about three and a half billion dollars a year—was to come out of the general revenues of the Treasury, and one-third out of deductions from the monthly Social Security checks received by those who voluntarily signed up. The A.M.A. pleaded with Byrnes not to submit his bill, arguing that it would drain away support for Eldercare. Since there was no support for Eldercare to speak of anyway, Byrnes went ahead and submitted his bill. The move was generally dismissed as a political grandstand play, and Byrnes himself privately conceded that the bill had no chance.

34

THE A.M.A.'s House of Delegates met on February 6th in a Chicago hotel called the Pick-Congress. Dr. Milford O. Rouse, now speaker of the house, opened the session by calling for "sober, optimistic, practical, dedicated enthusiasm and action." He refused afterward to tell reporters how much the action was going to cost. "We are not a wealthy organization," he said. "We have a modest reserve for a day just like this." The reserve was $14,735,000. The trustees denied reports that they were ready to spend four million dollars on the campaign, but it was then revealed that the A.M.A. had already distributed that sum to the state societies, which were expected to match it. One figure that was not in dispute was five hundred and fifty thousand dollars, which had been set aside, Dr. Ward announced, for newspaper, magazine, radio, and TV advertising. Shortly after the meeting, the Illinois Medical Society levied a special assessment on its members that raised a quarter of a million dollars, and a little later the Maryland Medical Society, also through a special assessment, raised a hundred and forty thousand dollars. When a member of the House Ways and Means Committee was told about these efforts, he smiled and said, "If we can rush Medicare through, we should be able to save the doctors several million dollars."

The A.M.A.'s strategy at that time was inspired by two recent events. The first was the publication early in January of a Gallup poll showing that although two-thirds of the people supported Medicare, forty per cent of them thought it covered *all* medical expenses. During the previous year, the A.M.A. had, more or less in passing, attacked Medicare on the ground that its coverage was inadequate, and now the Association began concentrating on this point, charging that the bill would take care of, variously, only twenty, twenty-three, or twenty-five per cent of the participants' medical expenses. The second event was Goldwater's unintentional success in scaring the wits out of older voters by his attacks on the Social Security system. An A.M.A. advertisement, fairly typical of thousands that soon appeared around the country, showed a pair of hands tearing a Social Security card in two, and warned "DON'T LET THIS HAPPEN TO YOU!" Below was the heading "Federal Medicare," followed by a description of its limited benefits, and, next to it, the heading "Doctors' Eldercare," followed by a description of its "unlimited" benefits, including coverage of all charges for hospitals, physicians, nursing homes, and drugs. The last line of the advertisement read, "A federal Medicare program could jeopardize your future through bankrupting the Social Security system."

This particular advertisement appeared widely in the home district of one of the co-sponsors of the Eldercare bill, Representative Herlong. Prompted by the National Council of Senior Citizens, some of the elderly among Herlong's constituents fl⌐ded him with angry letters; an old man in Ormond Beach, ⌐or example, asked, "Congressman, what aren't you capable of?" The National Council tipped off a reporter for United Press International about these letters, and he called Herlong, who promptly attacked the A.M.A. for making misleading statements. "For them to give the impression that [Eldercare] provides complete coverage is not so," he said. "It just makes it available for the states to provide it if they want to." Shortly after this interview appeared in Washington newspapers, one of the A.M.A.'s top officers and one of its chief lobbyists called on Herlong at his office. An hour later, Herlong issued a statement modifying what he had said earlier and attacking the Medicare forces for circulating "implied claims" about *their* bill.

The day after the A.M.A.'s House of Delegates wound up its special meeting in Chicago, Dr. Ward and several of his colleagues appeared before an executive-session hearing of the Ways and Means Committee. In the committee's earlier, public hearings, the chairman had indulged those witnesses, for both sides, who were clearly more interested in scoring debating points than in contributing to the committee's legislative purpose. But executive-session hearings were businesslike affairs. The committee was about to devise a bill, and its members wanted, and needed, all the expert assistance they could get on the complicated technical problems involved. In the invitations that Mills sent out to witnesses he specifically asked them to restrict their testimony to matters within their competence. All the witnesses complied except Dr. Ward and the A.M.A. officials accompanying him. They talked about economics, sociology, public welfare, and the Social Security system, and repeated, almost verbatim, the allegations made in their advertising. "The A.M.A. people had absolutely *nothing* constructive to offer," one member of the committee said afterward. "They spouted the usual nonsense, as if we were conducting a propaganda forum rather than a serious meeting. Then, when we indicated that we weren't interested, they got rude and ungentlemanly. Even Herlong and Curtis were annoyed. The behavior of the A.M.A. witnesses was the greatest favor that could have been done for the Medicare cause. Their refusal to coöperate relieved us of any obligation to them."

At one point during Dr. Ward's presentation of his prepared statement, he said:

We have seen a story in the February 1 issue of the St. Louis *Globe-Democrat* which quotes "an unpublished study by top government actuaries" and contains some rather ominous information, to state the matter mildly. According to the *Globe-Democrat,* the government actuaries have estimated that the cost of H.R. 1 would reach $3.8 billion a year by 1975, and, further, that the proposed special health-care fund would be just about broke by then. Let me quote . . . from the news story: "By 1975, according to the still secret study, the fund would be down to about $275 million. By 1976 the fund would be empty. What would happen then, in all probability, is that money would have to be diverted from the regular Social Security retirement fund to meet the Medicare deficits."

Representative Ullman, after saying, "I am only sorry that we must proceed in the writing of this bill without the technical assistance that your organization might have given us," proceeded to take up the *Globe-Democrat* story in some detail. "These are serious charges, and you simply don't bandy them around," he said to Dr. Ward. "Do you know where they came from?" Dr. Ward answered that he could get the reporter's name, since it was a byline story, and added that he would be "very happy to authenticate that statement." Ullman told him that it wouldn't be necessary. One reason Ullman and other members of the committee didn't feel that any further elaboration by the A.M.A. was necessary was that they already had a pretty good idea how the figures had found their way into print. A week earlier, Robert J. Myers, the chief actuary of the Social Security Administration, had appeared before the committee to answer various technical questions about the funding provisions of the King-Anderson bill. In the course of his testimony, Myers had used the figures that were later cited in the *Globe-Democrat* article, but he had used them as a hypothetical demonstration of the fact that health-care funds would be depleted by 1976 unless the taxable wage base was raised periodically—as the bill provided.

Having testimony taken by his own committee quoted back to him in a distorted form obviously angered Mills. "This was not secret information," he said to Dr. Ward. "This was information that I understand was obtained directly from Mr. Myers." Myers himself was in the room at the time, and Ullman asked him what had happened. It seemed that while Myers had not discussed the figures in question with any newspaper reporters, he had discussed them in some detail with other individuals. "The figures were obtained from my office by a representative of the American Medical Association, and they were from our worksheets," Myers said. When Dr. Ward left the witness chair, Mills watched him depart, and then turned to a colleague and said, "It's amazing. They haven't learned a thing."

35

AFTER the Committee on Ways and Means had heard the six-hundred-and-forty-first witness to appear before it since it opened its first hearings on the King-Anderson bill, in 1961, Mills announced in mid-February that the committee would begin to prepare the bill that would be sent to the floor of the House. Besides Medicare, Eldercare, the Byrnes bill, and a dozen other health-insurance measures that members of the House had submitted, the committee had before it an expanded and liberalized Kerr-Mills bill that Mills had introduced in the House in January and the amendment to the Social Security law providing a cash increase in pension benefits that had been deadlocked in the joint Senate-House conference committee the previous fall. Curtis and Herlong seemed rather embarrassed by Eldercare, and had little to say for it—so little, in fact, that they never brought it up for a vote. But Byrnes went all out for his contribution, which he began calling Bettercare. Byrnes's claim that his bill provided far more comprehensive coverage than any of the other bills made the Democrats uneasy, for although the Republicans might have no hope of getting the measure through Congress, they could be counted on to use it later as an example of how they had been trying to take care of old people when the Democrats betrayed them with a halfway piece of legislation. Mills had long been convinced that many people would be disappointed in Medicare—and angry at the administration that was responsible for it—when they found out how relatively little it gave them. Now, to make matters worse, the A.M.A.'s publicity on this point seemed likely to give organized medicine a we-told-you-so advantage in the consideration of any future legislation.

On the morning of March 2nd Mills called on Cohen, then H. E. W.'s Assistant Secretary for Legislation and now its Under Secretary, and asked him to give the committee a run-through of the various bills under consideration. At around three o'clock that afternoon, Cohen finished with the last of them—the Byrnes bill—and everyone looked at Mills to see what he would do next. No one was prepared for what happened. Turning to Byrnes, Mills said, "You know, John, I like that idea of yours"—the idea being Byrnes's plan for a voluntary program that the participants would help to pay for by agreeing to have small deductions taken from their monthly Social Security checks. As Mills continued, however, it became apparent that he liked the idea not as an alternative to Medicare but as a supplement to it. This arrangement, he explained, would provide a sort of three-layer cake: the expanded Kerr-Mills program making up the bottom layer, to take care of those close to indigence; Medicare making up the middle layer, to take care of the costs of hospital, nursing-home, and home-health care for the rest of the elderly; and the voluntary supplement making up the top layer, to take care of doctors' fees, in and out of hospitals. Then Mills turned back to Cohen and asked if the supplement could be made a part of the King-Anderson bill. Cohen quickly said that it could, and Mills asked him to draw up an amendment to that effect, along with an analysis of the costs, and adjourned the meeting until the following morning.

"Like everyone else in the room, I was stunned by Mills's strategy," Cohen said afterward. "It was the most brilliant legislative move I'd seen in thirty years. The doctors couldn't complain, because they had been carping about Medicare's shortcomings and about its being compulsory. And the Republicans couldn't complain, because it was their own idea. In effect, Mills had taken the A.M.A.'s ammunition, put it in the Republicans' gun, and blown both of them off the map." Byrnes, too, was stunned. "He just sat there with his mouth open," a member of the committee said later. Byrnes admitted after the meeting that Mills's maneuver had come as "quite a surprise" to him. "But, after all," he added, "the A.M.A. opened the door to all this with those advertisements."

President Johnson was also surprised, and amused, when he received a memorandum from Cohen describing the events of that afternoon and concluding, "The effect of this ingenious plan is . . . to make it almost certain that nobody will vote against the bill when it comes on the floor of the House." The President laughed, and said to the aide who had brought the note, "Just tell them to snip off that name 'Republican' and slip that little old amendment into the bill."

Early the next morning, a man from the A.M.A. appeared at the office of Representative Charles A. Vanik, a liberal Democrat from Ohio who was a new member of the Ways and Means Committee. Vanik wasn't in, but an assistant came out to the waiting room, and found the A.M.A. man slumped in a chair. The visitor asked if the rumor about Mills's coup was true, and upon being assured that it was he shook his head and got to his feet, with a dazed look. As he left, he said, "I never thought we'd end up spending several million dollars in advertising to expand the bill."

Cohen's presentation of the new plan before the Ways and Means Committee that morning took about half an hour. Myers had estimated that a contribution of three dollars a month by each participant, plus a matching sum from the Treasury—estimated at five hundred dollars the first year—would be sufficient to pay for eighty per cent of all the doctors' bills involved after each patient had paid a deductible of fifty dollars out of his own pocket. "O.K., it sounds fine," Mills said. That was all he said, and it was enough for the other members of the committee, who were used to accepting a casual remark from Mills as a final decision on even the most crucial matters. In effect, Mills had told them that he was adding the amendment to the bill—subject of course, to the committee's approval in a final vote.

Later in the day, Cohen discussed the new measure with

the President, who, he feared, might have had second thoughts about its added cost, since he was reported to be worried about the size of the forthcoming budget. Cohen told the President what the amendment would cost and outlined some of the political problems that this might present. When he had finished, the President nodded and asked what he could do to help. Somewhat puzzled, Cohen said that the basic question was whether the President could accept a five-hundred-million-dollar increase in the budget. As Mr. Johnson later recalled the conversation, he replied, "I'm going to run and get my brother." A good deal more puzzled, Cohen said he didn't understand. The President's explanation itself seemed cryptic, at first: "Well, I remember one time they were giving a test to a fellow who was going to be a switchman on the railroad, giving him an intelligence test, and they said, 'What would you do if a train was coming from the east going sixty miles per hour, and you looked over your shoulder and another one was coming from the west going sixty miles an hour, and they were heading for each other at just a mile separate? What would you do?' And the fellow said, 'I'd go get my brother.' And they said, 'Why would you get your brother?' And he said, 'Because he hasn't ever seen a train wreck.'" With that, the President told Cohen that he could have the five hundred million dollars, and warned him to watch out for trains.

A week later, on March 10th, two hundred members of the New York Golden Ring Council (which had been fighting for federal health insurance since the first Forand bill) went to Washington for a luncheon and rally in behalf of Medicare. By prearrangement with Mills, who had promised the Council action on Medicare the year before, the luncheon was held in the hearing room of the Ways and Means Committee. Next to the A.M.A., Mills had long been the chief villain of the Medicare drama in the view of many old people, but when he welcomed the members of the Golden Ring Council, they gave him a standing ovation. And when he told them that, as they had heard, the bill was to be greatly expanded, they gave him

189

another. "Mills is a politician of the first rank," William R. Hutton, of the National Council, said after the luncheon. "He anticipated the inevitable. He coöperated with the inevitable. And then he capitalized on the inevitable."

Being a realist, Mills expected the Republicans to accept the inevitable with comparable grace, since they could now turn the bill to their own advantage by claiming credit for a large part of it, but after the Golden Ring lunch he was told that Byrnes was talking about not voting for the bill, either in committee or on the floor. "He's got to," Mills said. "He's painted himself into a corner." But on March 23rd, when the Ways and Means Committee took a final vote on the bill (it was now being jocularly referred to in some quarters as Elder-Medi-Better-Care), Byrnes and all his fellow-Republicans voted against it, in a straight seventeen-to-eight party-line vote. The Democrats were jubilant. "I couldn't believe my ears when they voted no," one of them said. "Of course, Ford, the Minority Leader, had instructed them to. It was incredibly inept, politically. Now we'll get *all* the credit."

Leaving nothing to chance, President Johnson went on television at eleven o'clock on the morning of March 26th to describe the new bill. After giving a brief account of its provisions, he introduced nine other Democrats—from the House there were Mills, King, Speaker McCormack, Majority Whip Boggs, and Majority Leader Carl Albert, and from the Senate there were Anderson, Smathers, Majority Leader Mike Mansfield, and Byrd. All but Byrd spoke glowingly of the new measure—even Smathers said, "I'm delighted with the bill." Then the President turned to Byrd, who had opposed all the earlier, and far more modest, versions of the bill, and who, it was feared, as chairman of the Senate Committee on Finance, might hold up the present version by postponing hearings on it. In a dialogue that Representative Albert described later as not only an outstanding example of the famous "Johnson treatment" but the first instance of it ever to be shown on a national television hookup, the President smiled at Byrd and said, "I know that you will take an interest in the orderly

scheduling of this matter and giving it a thorough hearing."
Byrd looked at him blankly, whereupon Mr. Johnson asked,
"Would you care to make an observation?"

Byrd, who had engaged in many conversations with Presidents but never before with millions of people watching,
shook his head. "There is no observation I can make now,
because the bill hasn't come before the Senate," he replied
gruffly. "Naturally, I'm not familiar with it."

President Johnson pressed on. "And you have nothing that
you know of that would prevent [hearings] coming about in
reasonable time, not anything ahead of it in the committee?"
he asked.

"Nothing in the committee now," Byrd answered, shifting
uneasily.

"So when the House acts and it is referred to the Senate
Finance Committee, you will arrange for prompt hearings and
thorough hearings?" the President asked, leaning forward in-
tently.

Senator Byrd, in a voice that was barely audible, said,
"Yes."

Smiling broadly, Mr. Johnson banged his fist on the desk,
stared into the camera lens, and said, "Good!"

In a mood of high expectancy, the House met on April 8th
to vote on the first national health-insurance measure ever to
come before it. The Ways and Means Committee enjoys such
great prestige in the House, in large part because of the thor-
oughness with which it customarily conducts its business,
that the bills it reports out are rarely amended on the floor.
Instead, a period is set aside for description of the bill and for
debate on it, and then the opposition is permitted to recommend recommittal of the measure and its replacement by a
substitute. Mills received a standing ovation from both sides
of the aisle when he went to the rostrum in the well of the
House to describe what had by now become known as the
Mills bill. He quickly justified the reputation he had acquired
for always being in command of his material. Speaking without a trace of an accent—it is reported that he has an unusu-

191

ally strong one whenever he talks to a group of his constituents—and only rarely referring to notes, he outlined the provisions of the bill, which was two hundred and ninety-six pages long. The measure, he explained, included a seven-percent increase in pension benefits (thus breaking the tradition of keeping total Social Security taxes below ten per cent), an expanded Kerr-Mills program, a modification of the King-Anderson bill, and the Byrnes voluntary supplement. In all, the layer cake, with its cash frosting, was to cost about six billion dollars the first year—roughly half of it for health insurance. When Mills sat down, Byrnes presented his own original bill as the Republican alternative, and then for several hours members of both factions had their say. (Representative Herlong praised the Mills package.) When a vote was taken to send the Mills bill back to committee and substitute the Byrnes bill for it, it became clear that Mills's estimation of the situation the year before—that there wasn't enough support to get a Medicare bill through—had been right, for now the margin against the motion to recommit was only forty-five votes, or one more than the number of new Medicare advocates, both Democrats and Republicans, who were elected to the House in 1964. Sixty-three Democrats defected to Byrnes (Herlong among them), but only ten Republicans went over to the Medicare side. Once the recommittal vote was out of the way, however, and the Republicans were released from party discipline, the bill was approved by a vote of three hundred and thirteen (including Herlong) to a hundred and fifteen.

36

THE A.M.A.'s diagnosis had always been that once the body politic was infected by government health insurance, the illness would be irreversible. Although the patient was clearly on the point of succumbing by the spring of 1965, the A.M.A. prescribed another dose of its favorite medicine—a massive injection of publicity. Stepping up the campaign for Eldercare, the A.M.A. announced that the results of several polls showed the public to be heartily in favor of what the Association liked to call the Doctors' Program. At about that time, the A.M.A. sent every member of Congress a booklet of a hundred and seventy-one magazine-size pages containing "a cross-section of American editorial opposition to Medicare" and support for Eldercare. Anyone who took the trouble to glance through the compilation discovered that batches of the editorials were identical; for example, the same text appeared in the Birmingham *Post-Herald*, the Denver *Rocky Mountain News,* the Washington, D.C., *Daily News,* the Logansport, Indiana, *Press,* and the New York *World-Telegram & Sun.* Senator McNamara pointed out on the Senate floor that two of the editorials had appeared in ten different papers each, that another had appeared in eleven papers, and that six of the editorials had appeared in a total of fifty papers. The Association declared that McNamara had "slanted his remarks to imply editorials were sent out by the A.M.A.," and it denied the implied accusation. Shortly afterward, Morton Mintz, a top reporter on the Washington *Post,* traced some of the editorials in question to a couple of companies that specialized in preparing and distributing canned editorials. Neither of them charged the newspapers that used their services, but both charged those who wanted to have their views distributed; the A.M.A. was a client of both.

A little later, Senator Joseph D. Tydings, Democrat of Maryland, told his colleagues that his office, like theirs, had been flooded with mail—mostly form letters and form post-cards—attacking Medicare and praising Eldercare. Members of Congress usually ignore mail of this sort, but Tydings, who had been in the Senate only a few months, had conscientiously set about replying to more than ten thousand pieces of anti-Medicare mail with a two-page form letter of his own. He stopped before long, he said, because, of the first three hundred and fifty replies mailed out of his office, seventy-two came back marked "No such street," "No such street number," "Addressee unknown," or "Deceased." After Dr. Ward charged, in a speech before the Maryland State Medical Society around the same time, that Medicare would lead to government control of medical practice and would deprive patients of the right to choose whatever doctor they wanted, Walter F. Perkins, who for many years had been the president of the Johns Hopkins Hospital in Baltimore, told the press, "The American people are getting fed up with that sort of nonsense—and the members of Congress know it only too well."

Senator Byrd, having committed himself on television, scheduled the Finance Committee hearings on health-care legislation for late April. In fifteen days, the committee took more than twelve hundred pages of testimony, and heard scores of witnesses, among them the A.M.A.'s Dr. Ward. Apparently chastened by the reaction he had got from the Ways and Means Committee, Dr. Ward stuck quite closely this time to matters that fell within his competence as a physician. It was too late. The deference that was once shown to any representative of the medical profession who appeared before Congress had all but disappeared. In its place was outright derision—most openly displayed on this occasion by Senator Anderson, co-sponsor of the bill, who presided over many of the sessions, including the one at which the A.M.A. representatives appeared. Dr. Ward, in his opening remarks, brought up the Eldercare program, which he said had "aroused enthusiastic public support" and was the only measure providing medical care for the elderly that had been written "in consultation with the medical profession."

Senator Anderson broke in to list the names of a number of eminent physicians who had been consulted on the framing of the Medicare legislation, and then he asked whether the witness considered Dr. Benjamin Spock, whose name was on the list, a member of the medical profession. "If he has a Doctor of Medicine degree, yes," Dr. Ward answered. Sitting forward, Anderson asked sharply whether he meant to imply that Dr. Spock was not a licensed physician. Making amends, Dr. Ward said he was under the impression that Dr. Spock was a baby specialist. Anderson then produced a burst of laughter from the audience in the hearing room by inquiring whether Dr. Ward, a surgeon, was "an elderly specialist."

After a few more tart exchanges, Anderson asked if the A.M.A. objected to all forms of Social Security, including the monthly retirement check. Dr. Ward said that it did not, but Anderson pursued the subject.

> SENATOR ANDERSON: If you don't object to providing it for [the pensioner's] rent and other bills, why do you object to it for hospital bills?
> DR. WARD: In the first place, it should be based on need.
> SENATOR ANDERSON: Well, wait a minute. It isn't in the other case at all. If a man comes to the age of retirement and has a million dollars, he can draw his Social Security whether he needs it or not.
> DR. WARD: Yes, sir.
> SENATOR ANDERSON: You don't mind it as long as it isn't in your field.
> DR. WARD: No sir; I didn't say that.
> SENATOR ANDERSON: What *did* you say?
> DR. WARD: I object to the inclusion of people who are able to take care of themselves.
> SENATOR ANDERSON: These people in Social Security who paid their money over a period of time, they are allowed to draw their Social Security whether they need it or not. Do you object to that?
> DR. WARD: We have no argument about that.
> SENATOR ANDERSON: You don't object to that?

DR. WARD: We are concerned with health.

SENATOR ANDERSON: It is only when you get to your field that you object to it, isn't that right?

DR. WARD: After a fashion, yes, sir.

SENATOR ANDERSON: Thank you. I have no further questions.

The Finance Committee completed its hearings on May 19th and adjourned until the following week, when it was to go into executive working session to prepare its version of the House bill. The afternoon of the adjournment, Senator Long, who had won the post of Majority Whip (with Senator Anderson's help) after Hubert Humphrey became Vice-President, and who, after the death of Senator Robert Kerr, of Oklahoma, had become the ranking Democrat on the committee, held a press conference to announce that he intended to submit two amendments to the Mills package. The first of them, he said, would make Medicare's provisions unlimited, in order to take care of what he called "catastrophic illness." (Since a ten-minute illness can be catastrophic for the person suffering it, it was assumed that Long was using the term to describe long-term illnesses that were catastrophically expensive.) The second was designed to pay for this open-end feature by adding, on top of the increase in Social Security taxes, a sliding scale of deductibles, or amounts to be paid by the patients themselves, based on their incomes.

While the announcement came as a surprise to many people in Washington, it was clearly no surprise to the A.M.A., for the next issue of the *AMA News*, which had gone to press before Long called in the reporters, carried his description of the amendments. This set off speculation about whether the A.M.A. had developed the new program, but it turned out that Long had actually been contemplating such a plan for some time. As far back as the spring of 1963, he had mentioned the idea to Cohen, who was appalled by it for several reasons; namely, because it contained a means test (in the form of the deductibles based on income), because it was certain to be an administrative monstrosity, and because it was impossible to estimate how much it would cost, for, despite Long's assurances, there was no way of determining what would happen if hospitals were open to all comers for indefinite lengths of time.

In any event, Long did nothing further about his amendments during the first few weeks of the Finance Committee's executive-session deliberations. From time to time, he wandered into the room where the committee was meeting, and then, apparently deciding that the lineup of those on hand was unfavorable, explained that his duties as Whip required his presence on the floor, and departed. In the meantime, though, he talked privately with several of the liberal Democrats on the committee, assuring each of them in turn that his amendments, which none of them had yet seen, were nothing more than a reasonable expansion of the administration's bill. Since, as Whip, he was in some measure a representative of the administration, they assumed that he would not propose anything against the wishes of the President. Finally, late on the morning of June 17th, just as the committee was about to recess for lunch, Long appeared, looked around to see who was present and who was absent, and offered his amendments—not in the usual manner, by passing printed copies around, but by describing the details from his own copy. The amendments were far more extensive than he had indicated either in his press conference or in his private conversations with other senators.

In explaining his plan, Long repeated that it was merely an expansion of the administration's bill, and said that for a quarter of a billion dollars more they could provide unlimited hospital care for everyone sixty-five or over. He went on to warn his colleagues that the bill as it was currently written meant political disaster for all of them. The first time an old lady who had used up her allotted days of hospital care was carried out to die in the street, he said, there would be such a deafening public outcry that no senator who had voted for Medicare would ever be reëlected. Hurrying on, he told the committee that the scale of deductibles in his plan would be highly favorable to the poor, and described the breakdown— five per cent of the first thousand dollars of income, six per cent of the second thousand, and seven per cent of all income above that, with a minimum deductible of twenty dollars, and no maximum.

After a few minutes' discussion—representing perhaps the most casual treatment of a major piece of legislation in Senate history—Long called for a vote. The tally stood at seven to six for the amendments when Anderson, who had argued futilely against the plan, cast a proxy that had been given to him by Senator J. William Fulbright, of Arkansas. That made it a tie, and a defeat for Long. But Long broke in to say that he had a later proxy from Fulbright, and asked the committee's clerk to verify his claim. The clerk checked the date on Long's note from Fulbright and confirmed that it was more recent than the date on Anderson's. That made the vote eight to six for the amendments, and they were added to the bill. After the committee adjourned, Anderson, who was bewildered because he had been given Fulbright's assurance of support, asked the clerk for the proxy submitted by Long. When he examined it, he saw that it was indeed dated later than his but that it concerned another matter altogether.

In the Senate chamber that afternoon, Anderson told Fulbright about the incident, and together they confronted Long. "I thought this was supposed to be a gentlemen's club," Anderson said angrily. Long shrugged, said that perhaps there had been a misunderstanding, and offered to take another vote. Anderson, though he accepted the offer, did not accept the explanation—nor, it turned out, did many other senators, including Mansfield, who later gave Long a heated lecture on senatorial propriety at a Democratic policy meeting. Another proxy that had been misused—this one unintentionally—was one that Senator Albert Gore, Democrat of Tennessee, had given Senator Abraham Ribicoff, of Connecticut, over the telephone. Since Ribicoff had been a Medicare supporter all along, first as Secretary of the Department of Health, Education and Welfare under President Kennedy and then as a senator, Gore assumed that he would use the proxy in accordance with administration policy. Ribicoff, for his part, assumed that he was free to use it in accordance with his own best judgment, and he cast it for Long's amendments.

The two incidents produced a good deal of uncertainty all around. Senator Paul Douglas, of Illinois, who was the leading liberal in the Senate, had voted for Long's plan, but he began to have doubts about what he had done almost immediately. After the meeting broke up, he went back to his office and sat down to think things over. As a former professor of economics, he had no trouble working out the financial aspects of the bill, and he quickly figured out that only people with incomes less than eight hundred dollars a year (most of whom were already being cared for under existing welfare programs) would benefit more from the new bill than from the old one. As he also knew, the average hospital stay for those over the age of sixty-five was fifteen days. Perhaps most important of all, though, was his realization, he said later, that the Long proposal would "turn the nation's hospitals into warehouses for the senile." He added, "I saw that I had made a mistake. I simply hadn't understood the proposal." According to one high administration official, this may have been the first time in American history that a senator admitted he had been wrong.

On the morning of June 18th, the Cabinet met in a special session to discuss the situation in Vietnam. As the meeting got under way, Anthony Celebrezze, who had succeeded Ribicoff as Secretary of Health, Education and Welfare, said he was obliged to inform the President that there was a domestic crisis, and he explained what had taken place in the Finance Committee the previous day. The President jumped up and began pacing back and forth. "How could this have happened?" he demanded angrily. As soon as the meeting was over, he took steps to find out not only how it had happened but how it could be changed. Besides making telephone calls to the Democrats on the committee who had voted for the amendments without fully understanding their meaning, President Johnson called Long and appealed to him to withdraw his plan—without success. "I did not ask for this fight, but I do not run from one," Long told reporters. "I know the

White House is doing everything in its power to reverse the decision of the committee on my amendments. In my opinion, I will win."

In the view of several senators who had worked with Long over the years, winning was a complicated matter in this situation. If he couldn't stop the bill, they said, he intended to put his own stamp on it as clearly as Mills had put his. Moreover, having been compelled to go along with the administration on a civil-rights voting act, which had hurt him back in Louisiana, he was now publicly challenging the President as a way of showing his constituents that he was no Presidential errand boy. And, finally, Long was warning the White House that he couldn't be taken for granted. Whatever his motives may have been, he refused to discuss them in public. To one reporter who brought up the matter, he replied by launching into a forty-minute filibuster consisting largely of the A.M.A.'s favorite arguments—that Medicare was socialized medicine, that the British National Health Service was a failure, and that the labor movement supported the bill solely to save on its own welfare outlays. He also refused to explain why the only Republican on the committee who had supported him was Senator Carl Curtis, of Nebraska, an arch-conservative, who was generally considered to be the A.M.A.'s most ardent champion in the Senate now that Smathers had defected. All in all, Long appeared to enjoy the attention he was getting. He was reported to be especially amused by attacks on him in Northern newspapers, such as an editorial in the *Times* that took him to task for "acting in sublime disregard of his obligations as Democratic whip" and called his proposal "so disastrous that it is hard to believe it was put forward with any aim except to kill any prospect of Medicare in this session of Congress." In Louisiana, one senator later remarked, an attack by the *Times* hurts about as much as an attack by *Pravda*.

One of the key men on the committee was Senator Ribicoff, and in an attempt to persuade him to change his vote Cruikshank, of the A.F.L.-C.I.O., asked union members in Connecticut to let Ribicoff know that they strongly opposed the Long amendments. Then, a day or so later, Cruikshank went to see Ribicoff at his office.

The Senator jumped up and waved a sheaf of telegrams at Cruikshank. "What's all this?" Ribicoff demanded. "What do you mean by turning your people on me? You know I can't be pressured."

Cruikshank heard him out calmly, and then said, "You know, and I know, Abe, that if I came in here and you *hadn't* got all those wires, you wouldn't pay much attention to me." The issue, as Cruikshank saw it, was that the Long amendments were fiscally irresponsible, and he told Ribicoff that under no circumstances would the unions support any pie-in-the-sky scheme. Blue Cross, welfare assistance, and Social Security had limits, he said, so why shouldn't Medicare?

But the issue, as Ribicoff saw it, was humanitarian as well as political. "You don't have to walk along the street in New Britain, say, and have a constituent stop you and get sore because his dying mother was put out of a hospital after sixty days," he said. Besides, he went on, he supported only the open-end amendment, and not the deductible plan.

Cruikshank tried to convince Ribicoff that he couldn't support the first without also supporting the second, since the unlimited-care proposal had to be paid for. He got nowhere, and at the end of an hour each man stood where he had at the start.

The same day, a strategy meeting was held in Senator Douglas's office. The participants were, besides the Senator, Cruikshank; Cohen; Robert Ball, the Commissioner of Social Security; Leonard Lesser, Reuther's assistant; Mike Manitose, the White House liaison man with Congress; and Howard Bray, Anderson's assistant. Cohen and Ball had prepared a compromise proposal as a device in case something was needed to head off Long's amendments—a compromise that provided for sixty more days of hospital care (with a ten-dollar-a-day deductible to be paid by the patient) and a hundred and twenty more days of nursing-home care (with a five-dollar deductible). No one in the room liked the idea of a com-

201

promise, and when the subject came up, Douglas broke in to say that he would not agree to anything without first clearing it with Senator Anderson. Manitose was asked how the White House would react, and he said that the President would go along with whatever Anderson wanted. Then Cruikshank was asked about the A.F.L.-C.I.O's position. He said that he didn't like the idea of backing down. "But," he added, "we could live with it if we have to." As soon as the meeting broke up, Bray hurried off to tell Anderson about the proposal. Anderson's view was to decide the matter, and he refused to consider any compromise—at least, at that point. "We can keep it as a position to fall back to if we have to," he said. "But let's not do anything until we have to."

Later that afternoon, Cruikshank ran into a Democrat on the Finance Committee, Senator Vance Hartke, of Indiana, who shared Ribicoff's belief in the unlimited-care amendment offered by Long. Hartke flatly told Cruikshank that Anderson simply did not have the nine votes that were necessary to beat Long. Then, to Cruikshank's surprise and dismay, he mentioned the compromise plan and said that he was glad to hear that Cruikshank supported it. "I was shocked," Cruikshank recalled later. "I didn't know how much he knew." Hartke, it appeared, knew everything that had been said at the strategy meeting, for now he reminded Cruikshank, "You've already said you could live with it." With a nod, Cruikshank said, "Yes, but I also said I didn't like it." Ignoring this, Hartke went on to say that if Cruikshank would accept the compromise, he would personally guarantee ten votes for it, including Long's, and that by this means they could avoid a floor fight when the bill went to the Senate, which, he added, was otherwise inevitable. Cruikshank put him off with the reminder that he had no authority to alter the bill, and hurried off to see Anderson.

To Cruikshank's further dismay, he found that Anderson had left for the day and couldn't be reached. But he did reach Bray and told him that he had to see the Senator the first thing the following day, since the Finance Committee was due to meet at ten o'clock to take a new vote on the Long amendments. Promptly at nine the next morning—June 23rd—Cruikshank arrived at Anderson's office and told him about the leak from the strategy session of the previous day. As it happened, Anderson had had a similar experience with Hartke, who had also stopped him in the hall and said that he was glad to hear that Anderson supported the compromise. Feigning ignorance, Anderson had told Hartke that he knew nothing about any compromise, and had angrily assured him that he would not support one even if he did. Now Cruikshank asked whether they could be sure of nine votes, whereupon Anderson shook his head, explaining that he thought he had the nine but that he couldn't be certain. Anderson asked Cruikshank what they should do. After a pause, Cruikshank said, "Let's go for broke." Anderson broke into a smile and clasped his hand. "I hoped you'd say that," he said.

Meanwhile, the A.M.A.'s lobbyists were busy drumming up support for the bill as it had been amended by Long—not because they approved of it but because they saw in it a way to create a deadlock in the Senate-House conference committee, for everyone was convinced that Mills would never accept such a drastic change in his bill. The A.M.A. people had to move inconspicuously in this matter. For one thing, they could not openly support any legislation that set up a health-insurance program under Social Security, and, for another, they had become such political pariahs by this time that their support for a measure was apt to be a rather heavy burden. Not long before, an A.M.A. lobbyist, having learned that the A.F.L.-C.I.O. opposed the inclusion of chiropractors in the bill, since it felt, as the A.M.A. did, that they were not strictly medical practitioners, called a union lobbyist on the telephone and asked, "Can I announce that the A.M.A. and the A.F.L.-C.I.O are shoulder to shoulder on this?"

"No," the union man answered at once. "It's not a question of vengeance on our part," he went on. "It's a question of tactics. If you want to get something defeated in Congress, just say that the A.M.A. backs it."

There was a pause, and then the A.M.A. man said, "It's that bad?"

203

He was assured that it was.

The administration's strategists assumed that Long had originally avoided lining up the Republicans on the Finance Committee (except Curtis, who was believed to be working with him on the plan) because their support would have aroused the suspicions of the liberal Democrats, whom he needed far more. And now that the purpose of the plan had become clear it was also assumed that the rest of the Republicans, who hadn't understood the amendments the first time around any better than the Democrats had, would get behind Long in the hope that they could block Medicare. This assumption proved to be correct. When the committee met and a new vote was called for on the first of Long's amendments —the one adding a graduated deductible to the bill—all six of the Republicans sided with him, and all ten of the other Democrats, acceding to what the *Wall Street Journal* called "the administration's strenuous behest," voted against him. (Although Anderson had hoped for nine votes at best, Byrd unexpectedly sided with him, explaining that although he opposed Medicare on principle, he even more strongly opposed the unprincipled tactic of rendering a bill unacceptable and then submitting it to the Senate for a vote.) On the amendment providing unlimited care, two Democrats (Ribicoff and Hartke) who still liked the idea, behest or no behest, went over to Long, but two Republicans (Thruston B. Morton, of Kentucky, and Frank Carlson, of Kansas) went over to Anderson. That defeated both amendments. At once, Hartke proposed half of the compromise—that thirty days, with a ten-dollar-a-day deductible, be added. He explained that the deductible would keep the cost within reason, and in the end he prevailed. The following day, Long added the other thirty days of the compromise, and he, too, prevailed. As far as Anderson was concerned, this was a defeat, but a modest one. "The big thing," he said later, "was that we beat Long's openend scheme." With that settled, the committee voted out its version of the House bill by a final vote of twelve to five.

After the meeting broke up, several of the senators met with a group of reporters to explain the measure. Long had taken his defeat cheerfully, and he seemed to enjoy bantering with the newsmen, telling them that if they held off awhile the committee report would be ready as source material. "The staff is working on it right now," he said, and added, with a smile, "I guess we can dispense with the myth that senators write their own reports." He did not mention that the dissenting report he would submit was being written by a lobbyist for the A.M.A.

37

"AFTER nearly two decades of struggle and controversy, million-dollar advertising drives, rallies, and political-action campaigns, the A.M.A.'s crusade has failed," the *Medical World News* observed that June. "And in the opinion of many knowledgeable people in Washington, the A.M.A.'s own strategy of uncompromising resistance contributed to the dimensions of its defeat." As if those dimensions weren't broad enough already, the A.M.A. now laid out still more money on still another public-relations push. Before June was over, it had placed a large advertisement entitled "An Open Letter to Our Patients" in a hundred major newspapers around the country. A week after that appeared, it put on nationwide television a half-hour program called "Health Care at the Crossroads." And its members continued to pour letters and telegrams by the thousand onto the desks of congressmen, urging them to oppose any interference by the government with what the medical profession had traditionally regarded as its own "sacred trust" of caring for the sick.

On June 20th, some twenty-five thousand doctors arrived in New York for an A.M.A. convention, and were met by five hundred elderly pickets who handed out leaflets entitled "An Open Letter to Our Doctors." The opposition that had arisen at the previous convention among doctors who felt that the A.M.A. was going too far was now drowned out by outcries from doctors who felt that it wasn't going far enough. Six weeks earlier, the Ohio State Medical Association, representing ten thousand doctors, had approved a resolution calling on its members to refuse to take part in any federal health-insurance program. Shortly after that, the right-wing Association of American Physicians and Surgeons sent a letter to every doctor in the country stating that "now is the time for you and every other ethical physician in the United States to individually and voluntarily pledge nonparticipation in . . . the socialized hospitalization and medical care program for the aged." The delegates in New York seemed to be strongly in favor of a boycott. Dr. Ward, in his speech as outgoing president, told them, "One poll after another has demonstrated beyond question that the American people have the most serious misgivings about welfare statism," and he received tumultuous applause.

When Dr. James Z. Appel, the incoming president, warned the assemblage against "unethical tactics such as boycott, strike, or sabotage" and said that doctors should defy neither the letter nor the spirit of any law passed by Congress, he got a very different reaction. He was accused of being responsible for "appeasement," "surrender," and the destruction of "the American dream." In the convention's first session on legislative matters, nine state delegations—from Arizona, Ohio, Florida, Texas, Indiana, South Carolina, Connecticut, Nebraska, and Louisiana—introduced separate resolutions calling for a boycott. When the House of Delegates' Committee on Legislation and Public Relations heard testimony on the boycott resolutions, only a few physicians stood by Dr. Appel. The view of the majority was perhaps expressed most eloquently by a delegate from New Jersey who told the committee, "Force must be used when reason will not prevail."

Actually, a number of A.M.A. members and officials, including most of the trustees, saw danger in the headlong rush toward a boycott. Apparently they were aware that the medical profession had lost a good part of the public respect it had once commanded, and, further, that a concerted refusal to obey a law of the land might push Congress to take even more drastic action. In any case, everyone expected the issue to be resolved by the delegates' designation of a president-elect, to be installed the following summer. The two leading contenders for the post were Dr. Charles L. Hudson, of Ohio, who opposed his state medical society's boycott resolution, and Dr. Durward G. Hall, of Missouri, a Republican member of Congress, who had openly campaigned for a boycott. The trustees had always had their way in the past, and they had it this time, too—after they had rounded up enough votes to elect Dr. Hudson. Though Hudson was an avid Goldwater fan ("I'm still unhappy he didn't win," he said), he was a moderate in the A.M.A. After his election, and the investiture of Dr. Appel, the delegates accepted a recommendation by the trustees that they sidestep the boycott question by reaffirming the Association's previous policy declarations in general terms. By this time, most of the advocates of uncompromising resistance had been calmed down. "Only one doctor rose on the floor in favor of a boycott," Robert C. Toth of the Los Angeles *Times* reported, "but he tried to illustrate his point with a joke about an unwed Negro mother, which did nothing to help his cause." The delegates also rejected a resolution, submitted by the Oregon delegation, that would have given the A.M.A.'s endorsement to the Surgeon General's report on the dangers of smoking.

38

When the fog of partisan oratory over a controversial measure before Congress finally thins out and the road of political necessity appears ahead, legislators usually find that a bandwagon is the most comfortable vehicle to ride on. The House Medicare bill emerged from the Senate by a vote of sixty-eight to twenty-one and with five hundred and thirteen amendments and a billion and a half dollars in costs added to it. In part, the Senate's access of generosity was due to its members' awareness that they could claim credit for trying—as in a third-of-a-billion-dollar amendment, submitted by Hartke, to assist the blind, in which the definition of blindness was broad enough to include poor eyesight—but could confidently rely on the Senate-House conferees to behave responsibly and eliminate the unnecessary embellishments. Byrd had appointed Long to serve as the floor manager of the bill, and by the second day of the three-day debate so many amendments had been loaded on that the administration began to suspect that some of the Senators were deliberately trying to make the bill unacceptable to the House conferees. Accordingly, the President asked Long not to consider any but essential amendments from that point on, whereupon Long went to the floor and called for more amendments.

To many of those watching the performance, it seemed that Long, having been beaten in the Finance Committee, was carrying his fight to the floor of the Senate. As a matter of fact, he had entered into an agreement not to do that. The news of his initial success in putting his amendments through the committee had irritated one of his more influential and resourceful constituents, a labor leader in Louisiana, to whom

209

Long had previously given his word that he would support Medicare down the line. Moving quickly, the man made arrangements to block action on a tax-write-off bill on oil holdings that was then being considered by a committee of the state legislature and that had been written expressly for the Longs, whose money was largely in oil. When Long heard about this maneuver, he telephoned the union leader and asked him what he thought he was doing. "What do you think you're doing to Medicare?" the man demanded. In the end, the labor leader agreed to release the tax bill in exchange for Long's agreement to confine his fight against Medicare to the Finance Committee. True to his word, Long did not carry his fight to the floor of the Senate. He let others carry it there for him. When he openly supported the amendments he had originally proposed, and failed to line up votes for the administration's position, Anderson said to Mansfield, "My God, Mike, we've got a floor manager who's against the bill!"

Senator Curtis submitted Long's amendment for graduated deductibles, which was by now almost universally interpreted as a maneuver, in behalf of the A.M.A., to create a stalemate when the conference committee met. There were certain ironies in the situation, both for Curtis and for the A.M.A., since the amendment was clearly aimed at soaking the rich. Under its provisions, those who paid the most into the Social Security fund during their working years would get the least out of it for medical care after they retired. In large part because Long had failed to explain the administration's policy to the members of his party, the amendment came within ten votes of being passed. An administration official who was asked whether the narrow margin might not encourage Curtis to reintroduce the amendment in another form said, "No, that would be too dirty. It was offered for a vote and beaten fairly." The next day, Curtis did reintroduce it in another form, and again it lost.

Long's other amendment—for unlimited hospital care—was offered by Senator Ribicoff, who made an impassioned plea for it, as Long nodded and smiled. Anderson and Douglas had done their best to persuade Ribicoff that he was endangering the entire Medicare program, but he had gone ahead anyway. After taking a head count, Mansfield told his colleagues that they couldn't hope to beat the amendment. The prediction upset Anderson so much that he became ill and was forced to take to his bed. During the debate, several liberal senators who were uncertain about which way they should vote were told that the A.F.L.-C.I.O. was behind the amendment. When the story reached Cohen, who was on hand outside the chamber, he rushed to a telephone and called Cruikshank to ask if it was true. Cruikshank said it wasn't, and hurried over to the Capitol, where he found Douglas and Gore trying to rally the Medicare forces, and told them where the unions stood. Douglas and Gore passed the word around, and then Mansfield arose to deliver a rebuttal to Ribicoff that Anderson had been scheduled to give before he became ill. The speech, which, Anderson himself publicly said later, had been written by Cruikshank, turned the tide—or at least so Ribicoff said afterward. The quality of the speech itself and the authority it bore because of Mansfield's position as the administration's spokesman finally won over enough senators to defeat Long—but only by four votes.

One of the last issues to be raised before the final vote was taken on the bill was whether doctors should be put under the Social Security system. At that time, they were the only major professional group not covered. Polls conducted by state medical societies showed that a majority of the country's physicians wanted to be included in the program, but the A.M.A., which had refused over the years to poll its members nationally on the question, opposed their inclusion. Just before the vote on the amendment, Gore rose to say, "The A.M.A. has made such a fine contribution to the enactment of Medicare that I think it has earned the right to come under its benefits." Amid general laughter, the proposal was approved, and shortly after that, on July 9th, so was the entire bill.

39

As had been expected, Mills lopped a great chunk off the Senate measure when the conference committee met—one and a quarter billion dollars, in fact. One of the major differences between the House and Senate bills concerned the way four categories of specialists—pathologists, radiologists, anesthesiologists, and physiatrists (physical therapists)—were to be paid. The measure that Mills reported out of the Ways and Means Committee transferred the arrangements for paying these doctors from the Medicare, or hospital, section of the act to the voluntary-insurance supplement. Most of the specialists in the four categories either worked on salaries at hospitals or billed the hospitals for their work, though some of them did bill patients directly. This last method was the least common and the most costly, but the Mills provision would make it standard for millions of elderly patients, and hospitals would lose control over fees for even the most routine procedures. The A.M.A. backed Mills on this point—it had always opposed the idea of doctors' working on salary—and the specialists themselves insisted that they should be treated like other doctors, not like mere technicians.

"Although the arguments have largely revolved around ethics and patient care, the issues have almost inevitably ended up in dollars," Dr. Albert W. Snoke, the executive director of the Grace-New Haven Community Hospital and a former president of the American Hospital Association, wrote Mills in a letter complaining about alterations that had been made in the King-Anderson bill. Dr. Snoke argued that once the four kinds of specialists were free to charge what the traffic would bear, the costs to patients and hospitals would skyrocket, and the ultimate consequence, he said, would be total government control.

Naturally, the President didn't want to be held responsible for supporting a program that was certain to raise medical costs, so he instructed Cohen to see if he could persuade Mills to change his mind. Cohen got together with Mills, McCormack, Albert, and Boggs in the office of the Speaker of the House to try to work something out, but when McCormack picked up the telephone to call the President, Mills—apparently unwilling to be subjected to the Johnson treatment—quickly left the room. His decision, he later told an administration official, was political and was not open to negotiation. After the bill reached the Senate floor, Douglas pointed out that the administration had promised all along that it would not interfere with medical practice in any way, and that as the bill stood it did interfere, since it told hospitals how their doctors had to be paid. To rectify this, Douglas offered an amendment that would leave it up to the hospitals to decide how the specialists were to be paid. At the urgent request of the President, Secretary Celebrezze, the American Hospital Association, and hundreds of hospitals and doctors around the country, the Senate accepted the Douglas amendment.

In the conference, Mills led the administration to believe that he was ready to compromise on the issue, and Cohen thereupon prepared an amendment that excluded from the Medicare section of the law only the anesthesiologists, who often billed patients directly anyway, and the physiatrists, whose bills were not expected to constitute a large financial problem. But when the time came for a vote, Mills held out for the House position, and Boggs, who in the past had always stuck by the administration on Medicare, did, too. After no resistance at all, Long and Smathers joined their Republican colleagues in supporting Mills's position, and the compromise plan was defeated. "It was obviously prearranged," one of the other Senate conferees said afterward. "Mills had promised the doctors that he would never put any of them under any compulsory system, and he kept his word. Unfortunately, it's going to cost the American people hundreds of millions of dollars. It's also going to make a hopeless mess out of normal hospital procedures. The President has asked us to repeal the

213

amendment, so we'll just have to start fighting all over again."

The final form in which Medicare was reported out of conference on July 26th was far more comprehensive than any of the bills that had led up to it. The bill provided every person sixty-five or older—except retired federal employees, who are covered by the Federal Employees Health Benefits Act—with sixty days of free hospital care, after a standard forty-dollar deductible to avoid unnecessary hospitalization; thirty more days of hospital care at a charge of ten dollars a day (a compromise on the Hartke-Long Compromise); twenty days of free nursing-home care; eighty more days of nursing-home care at a charge of five dollars a day (ditto); a hundred home visits by nurses or other health specialists after hospitalization; and eighty per cent of the cost of hospital diagnostic tests, after a twenty-dollar deductible for each series. To pay for this, the taxable wage base of the Social Security system was raised to sixty-six hundred dollars a year, and the tax itself was increased by one-half of one per cent for both employee and employer. (Because of Mills's insistence that the program be doubly sound actuarially, the increase was double the amount proposed in the bill of the year before.) The voluntary supplement provided for payment of eighty per cent of what the bill called "reasonable charges" for all physicians' services, after a fifty-dollar-a-year deductible; another hundred home health visits, whether a patient had been hospitalized or not; and the costs of non-hospital diagnostic tests, surgical dressings, splints, and rented medical equipment. To pay for this coverage, people sixty-five or older who wished to participate were to contribute three dollars a month apiece, and their contributions were to be supplemented by a matching sum from the Treasury's general revenues—both amounts being subject, as were the other cost-sharing provisions, to revision in future years if costs rose appreciably. After more than fifty years of debate on whether the United States should adopt a national health-insurance program and, if so, what form it should take, this complex but typically American solution to the problem was passed by the House on July 27th and by the Senate on July 28th.

40

IN ORDER to discuss the application of Medicare, the A.M.A. requested an appointment with the President, and on July 29th he met with eleven of its leaders at the White House. "I'd never seen anything like it," one of the administration officials who attended the meeting said afterward. "The President made a powerful, moving appeal to the doctors to accept the new law, and reminded them that it had been devised after long and thorough consideration by the people's representatives under our constitutional procedures. He went on in that way for some time, and then he began talking about what wonderful men doctors were, and how when his daddy was sick the doctor would come over and sit up all night with him, and charge a pittance. He was getting terribly corny, but he had them on the edge of their seats. Then, suddenly, he got up and stretched. Of course, when the President of the United States stands up, everybody stands up. They jumped to their feet, and then he sat down, so they sat down, too. He started off again, with another moving statement about this great nation and its obligation to those who had helped make it great and who were now old and sick and helpless through no fault of their own. Gradually, he moved back to the cornfield, and then he stood up again, and again they jumped to their feet. He did that a couple more times—until they were fully aware of who was President—and then he turned to a memorandum on his desk. He read them the statement in the bill prohibiting any government interference in any kind of medical practice at any time, and also the statement guaranteeing freedom of choice for both doctors and patients, and assured them there would be no government meddling in these matters. Next, he explained that Blue Cross and private insurance carriers, who are the administrative middlemen under the law, would determine the bill's definition of 'reasonable charges' on the basis of what was customary for a given area. Naturally, the doctors went for this, because they have great influence with most of those outfits. Toward the end, he asked for their help in drawing up regulations to implement the law. Then he got up one last time, and said that he had to leave. Before he went, he turned to Cohen, who is the A.M.A.'s idea of an archfiend, and, shaking a huge forefinger in his face, he said, 'Wilbur, I want you to stay here with these gentlemen, and work things out according to my instructions—no matter how long it takes you.' Afterward, I overheard one A.M.A. man say to another, 'Boy, did you hear how he talked to Cohen?' Of course, Wilbur had written the memorandum."

The day after the conference with the doctors, President Johnson flew out to Independence, Missouri, to sign Public Law 89-97 at the Harry S. Truman Memorial Library. Although by this time the A.M.A.'s leaders had apparently seen the futility of continued opposition, they were finding it almost impossible, after years of doing their best to stir up their members, to calm them down. In fact, boycott fever among doctors had reached epidemic proportions. The Association informed its members that while its lawyers had advised it that any concerted boycott might constitute a violation of the antitrust laws, individual doctors were free to refuse on their own to participate in the program. The statement obviously ran counter to Dr. Appel's plea for moderation and for obedience to the laws of the land, but it still didn't satisfy the more militant A.M.A. members. The Association of American Physicians and Surgeons accused the A.M.A. of "an indefensible display of collaboration with and complicity in evil," and appealed by mail to all doctors to join it in a boycott, concerted or not. Dr. Annis estimated that ninety per cent of all the physicians in the country would refuse to touch a government form. It was also reported that some doctors urged their elderly patients not to sign up for Medicare, and told them that if they did, they would have to find another physician.

By early fall, the pressure for a strike against the law had become so nearly irresistible that the A.M.A., in response to petitions from its state societies, called a special session of the House of Delegates. At the meeting, which was held in Chicago at the beginning of October, Dr. Annis told the delegates, to resounding cheers, that Medicare had been "passed by every mockery of the Democratic process," and that the nation's physicians had been betrayed by "appeasers," "collaborators with the enemy," "labor bosses," and "power-hungry political leaders." He did not recommend a boycott, however. Instead, he declared that the A.M.A. should coöperate with the government and get "inside the camp of the enemy" in order to "find the vital, the vulnerable spots." Dr. Annis's views carried a good deal of weight, and in the end they prevailed. Still, a number of delegates threatened to conduct personal boycotts, and several of them said they would go to jail before they would coöperate in any way with the government. Actually, there was no way for them to carry out this threat short of forcing their way into jail, for the law provided that if a doctor refused to fill out a Medicare form and, instead, sent his bill to the patient as usual, the patient could collect from the government by simply sending in the doctor's bill and a record of its having been paid. Before long, the determination to bill patients directly became a movement of some size among doctors. It was led by Dr. Annis, and it was considered by many people in the government to be largely obstructive, since for many years doctors had been filling out patients' forms for Blue Cross, Blue Shield, and other insurance programs.

Dr. Appel—by now the voice of moderation in the Association—was not warmly received when he rose and told his colleagues that they were "expected by the public, the press, and the Congress to act as reasonable and mature men and women." And the response was even cooler when he said, in conclusion, "I submit . . . that no political crisis is as deleterious to medicine as one brought about by its members."

Not long afterward, Senator Douglas, who had become Congress's unofficial overseer of the Medicare program, submitted several bills to amend the law—chief among them an amendment that returned the four specialist groups to the hospital-coverage part of the plan. Along with many other members of Congress who had fought for government health insurance over the years, he was increasingly upset by the doctors' threats to boycott or in one way or another sabotage the Medicare program. "We've had a lot of reports about doctors planning to raise their fees so that the 'reasonable charges' prevailing in their area would be higher," the Senator said. "Of course, as soon as the bill was passed, they said it would never work and that the administration would be to blame for its failure. We'll know where the blame lies—and so will the people. The doctors of this country say they have a sacred trust. I hope they keep it."

Index

228